heartfelt manner. There will always be challenges that surround us and I feel blessed to know there is someone out there such as Pat!"

–Dave Pelzer, National Jefferson Award Recipient, former CA Fire Captain, *New York Times* best-selling author of *A Child Called "It"* and *Return to the River*

"From the skies above Pennsylvania to the streets of Detroit, a British cancer ward, and more, the stories in *Bump in the Road* will engage and inspire you to overcome any obstacle that comes your way. It's a gem of a book that I absolutely loved."

–Kristen Carter, Metastatic Breast Cancer (MBSC) Leadership Team, breast cancer advocate and coach

Praise for
Bump in the Road: Stories of Courage, Hope and Resilience

"This is a beautiful book about life, its imperfections, its challenges, and its joys. It is a book of hope and wisdom for all of us facing a bump in the road."

–Pragito Dove, author of #1 Amazon best-selling *Lunchtime Enlightenment: Expressive Meditations for Manifesting Peace, Prosperity, and Passion*

"Pat has woven together beautiful stories of life setbacks that have been transformed into spiritual growth. This book is a gift and a must-read for souls experiencing pain and yearning for growth."

–Gary Hensel, author of the Best-Selling Book *Lessons For A Spiritual Warrior*

"It is easy to find the personal in the general; it is quite another thing to find the general in the personal. Pat Wetzel has done that for us. Like the Zen Master in chapter 24, she has shown us how to fill ourselves with wisdom with personal stories with which we all can identify."

–Bill Aron, author and photographer

"We are taught as we grow up about what impresses others but not about how to find our way and live our lives. When you know where you are going, the bumps are nonexistent or meaningless and cannot stop our moving forward and living a full life."

–Bernard Siegel, MD, author of *Love, Medicine & Miracles, Prescriptions For Living* and *365 Prescriptions for The Soul*

"Pat Wetzel's *Bump in the Road* recounts so many lives of personal challenge and subsequent growth. Through these remarkable stories, Pat shares bumps in the road and bumps in the air too. Her stories illuminate the journey of the human soul and invite the reader to learn from her stories and others so that we may all find some lift and soar to our highest levels."

–Terry Chase, ND, MA, RN, speaker-consultant-author, *Spoke by Spoke: How a Broken Back and a Broken Bike Led to a WholeHearted Life*

"A wonderful book full of heart speak. A good reminder that life is happening right now, right here . . . don't miss it!"

–Nick Adkins, Co-Founder and Board Member, PinkSocks

"Pat is a beautiful human being and has written a beautiful book, full of wonderful, inspiring, and insightful stories. You are so going to enjoy reading it."

–Manoj Krishna, Founder of The Human Wisdom Project

"Pat Wetzel has woven together a rich tapestry of memoir and others' personal accounts of navigating and conquering some massive bumps in life's paths. The stories grab you from beginning to end, and then cling to you long after you close the book. This is the ultimate motivator and guide for someone who has been blindsided by traumatic change in their life."

–Cameron Auxer, author of *When Bodies Break: How We Survive* and *Thrive with Illness and Disability*

"Pat Wetzel has crafted a guide for life's toughest times. The roughest moments really are infuriatingly effective in accelerating our personal and spiritual growth! We don't like it, don't want it, and are threatened by it . . . yet troubling times wake us up to what is most important, and even more, to what we are, which is more magnificent than we can imagine. The struggles have so much energy for transformation, so let's not only go through them but grow through them. Don't waste the crisis!"

–David Maginley, M.Div, CSCP, chaplain, author, public speaker

"In the course of a life, one never knows what events may transpire. Pat Wetzel has literally dedicated her life's work in the service of others. *Bump in the Road* is written for the sole purpose of helping all of us in a calming,

BUMP IN THE ROAD

15 STORIES OF **COURAGE, HOPE** AND **RESILIENCE**

PAT WETZEL

Published by Serendipity Press
www.BumpInTheRoad.us

ISBN (paperback): 979-8-9887954-0-7
ISBN (ebook): 979-8-9887954-1-4

Book design and production by www.AuthorSuccess.com

To all my podcast guests who have so generously shared their wisdom and stories to help the rest of us navigate life's bumps.

DISCLAIMER

No part of this book should be construed as medical or psychological advice. Some details have been altered to provide a more coherent time frame or to obscure the identity of certain individuals. In some stories, time has been compressed to present a coherent chronology. The transcripts are all edited.

A GIFT TO MY READERS

FOR YOU, MY DEAR READER, A GIFT!

There is so much more to explore in *Bump in the Road*, including a private Reader's Portal where you'll find more about each guest including unedited conversations, videos, and photos. There's also a Workbook.

These resources can be found at BumpInTheRoad.us/Readers-Portal/ or by scanning the QR code below. Enjoy!

Contents

Introduction

What have I done?

I sold my perfect house. I'm about to hit the road with no idea where I'm going. And more importantly, I have no idea where this little foray might lead.

Road trips are a habit of mine. Travel is a remnant from my early years. My family spent months overseas; I grew up exploring new towns and cities where I didn't speak the language or know the customs.

I got hopelessly lost in Paris. My cousin deserted me on a French beach, and I had to find my way back to the villa via twisting cobblestone streets dating back to the Romans. In Czechoslovakia, I couldn't read the road signs. In Greece, I simply pointed to a large roast on a roadside rotisserie.

I am grateful for those early experiences because they set the tone for much of what was to come.

Those experiences taught me to follow my intuition. To be curious. To trust in myself and to go forward in uncertainty and even fear. I learned to see life as an adventure.

And that is something we all must learn to do.

We're all on our own road trip. You must ask yourself, are you happy? Are you living the life you dreamed about?

Perhaps you want more meaning. Perhaps you want more love or connection. Perhaps you simply want to be happier.

Whatever it is you seek, I guarantee that you already know the answers. The answers lie within.

The journey within is the greatest adventure you'll ever take. It's an intangible world full of discovery, truth, and wisdom. It's about revelation and transformation. And a few bumps. Because everyone hits a bump in the road.

I've traveled a long and sometimes bumpy road, from corporate life to disability, from marriage to divorce, from seeking something outside myself to finding peace within. Along the way I've become passionate about stories that touch our souls and change our lives.

Stories create a shared moment of connection, and in that moment, we are one. We feel a mutual understanding, compassion, and perhaps wisdom. That shared emotion is a moment that can connect and change us.

It is said that the personal is universal. Come share the personal stories of my guests, because their story *is* your story. Their hurdles *are* yours. And their wisdom and insight can be yours, too.

The Birth of "Bump"

The idea for *Bump in the Road* (which I affectionately refer to as "Bump") was born out of upheaval. Covid shut down a project, CancerRoadTrip, I had been working on for over two years, wiping out the corporate sponsorships I'd worked so hard to line up, as well as my own investment in both time and money. CancerRoadTrip was a film and travel project which told the stories of people impacted by cancer against the backdrop of exotic travel. Think Kilimanjaro and the metaphor of a mountain. Think safari and the metaphor of survival. Think Zanzibar and the spice of life.

When the world shut down in 2020, so did CancerRoadTrip; and so did I. Large bags of salty potato chips became my food of choice when facing the total, cataclysmic, unwanted uncertainty that appeared before me. I knew I needed to move forward; but forward to what? My project was gone. My investment was gone. The future was highly unknown on so many levels.

I decided to launch a podcast. Physical travel may have shut down, but I could still travel the globe virtually.

But what would I talk about? What inspired me?

I have always been inspired by adventure. I love to travel and explore. "The Road" and the search for an authentic life is an integral part of my story. In a moment of intuition and inspiration, I named the podcast *Bump in the Road*. Feeling lost, I was wondering where do I find the wisdom to navigate this adventure called life? What is my true north? What can I learn from others? And I turned to my podcast guests for guidance.

Facing uncertainty, my podcast guests have transformed their lives. Each of them dared to take the road less traveled, and in doing so found a truth, *their truth*, that changed everything.

Daring to Live an Authentic Life

Every week on my podcast *Bump in the Road*, my guests share stories of how they've navigated their life's detours. Everyone's story is unique, but the themes are the same. They are universal themes of the human journey: challenge, hope, triumph, courage, and more.

In reading this book, pick a chapter that speaks to you. The chapters can be read in any order.

All the chapters are structured in the same way:

- An overview
- A story from my life paralleling the chapter theme
- An introduction to my guest
- An edited transcript of our conversation, followed by some "thoughts for you to ponder" and some "key takeaways."

For my readers, there's also a free multi-media reader's portal that includes a workbook as well as videos, subscriber-only podcasts (all free to you), photos, and more about each guest. You can access all this here:

Or just visit BumpInTheRoad.us/Readers-Portal

Five Steps to a Meaningful and Authentic Life

In the last section of the book, *Five Steps to a Meaningful and Authentic Life,* I offer some thoughts for living your best life. These concepts are timeless. They will serve you through good days and bad; they will help you look within to find your true north. They will help you find how to:

- Develop the mental flexibility to embrace change
- Find your authentic self
- Let go of that inner voice that holds you back
- Cultivate conscious thought
- Find your unique purpose

If there is one takeaway from all the stories in this book, it is that life is an adventure and you are not alone. Everyone hits a bump in the road. The question becomes, what do you choose to do with it?

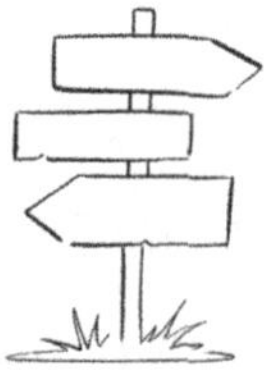

PROLOGUE

The Start of it All

1993

There is a private airfield in Pennsylvania near the Maryland border. At the entrance is a sign: **Private Property No Trespassing. Go away**, it warns in no uncertain terms.

Runways, hangars, a fuel depot, and a somewhat dilapidated control tower look out over acres of green grass, tarmac, and trees. The trees bend with the wind, the old hangar door creaks, and an orange windsock moves this way and that, chasing the energy of the air.

Had I heeded that warning to "Go away," I would not be here. But I am, and today is my first flight in my new plane. I am excited, proud, and nervous.

I'm also terrified.

Sweat forms on my brow. Under my flying hat, the moisture is plastering my naturally wavy hair into a heavy, lifeless mat. The weight of a big, ungainly parachute tilts me backwards. The leg straps are so tight I can barely walk.

I waddle towards the plane with trepidation. Several pilots stand by the aircraft, holding the wing, removing the rear wheel dolly used to transport the plane on the tarmac, and preparing the launch. For them, it's just another day, another plane, another launch. For me, it's a moment of fear laced with possibility.

As I approach the tarmac, it is my fear that envelopes me. I feel as though I am passing through a portal, like in a science fiction novel. The passage might be dangerous, or it might be benign. It might lead to a black hole; it might open brilliant new worlds. But I must push through it to see what lies on the other side.

My fear is twofold. First, this is a high-performance, single-seat sailplane with five flap settings and retractable gear. No one can teach me how to fly it. I simply must do it. There is no engine and no go-around. I have one shot to get it right.

This plane also has a bit of a reputation, both for speed and for some violent behavior. Several very experienced pilots died in this type of aircraft. I am not very experienced, and I am afraid that may be my own fate, as well. Or so the old pilot who ran the airport on the ridge told me when he heard about the plane I had purchased.

"You're going to kill yourself in *that plane,*" he declared.

I'd rented a plane to get some experience ridge flying. Ridge flying is when you trade the energy of an approaching weather front as it collides with a mountain ridge for distance and speed.

I nailed my landing on a wild and windy day. I was proud of my flight. But the old pilot who owned the airfield sauntered up to me and informed me that my soon-to-be new plane was way out of my league.

My excitement over my perfect landing on a wild and windy day abruptly vanished, replaced by a sinking feeling in the pit of my gut. What if the old pilot was right?

Those words become a not-so-subconscious mantra that plays over and over in my head. And now, today, I am making my first flight in *that plane* with everyone at the airfield watching.

Balancing the bulky parachute on my back, I awkwardly swing one leg, then the other, over the side of the plane and settle into the pilot's seat. I stretch out my legs towards the rudder pedals and adjust the seat. Even though I've spent hours poring over the manual, sitting in the cockpit, and developing detailed checklists, everything feels alien.

This is the first time I've sat on the runway in preparation for taking off. From the semi-reclined position, I realize that I can barely see over the instrument panel. The cockpit is built for a large man; I am a small woman. One of the pilots, a Navy test pilot, shoves a piece of Styrofoam behind my back to help me sit up and see beyond the panel of dials and indicators.

I learned to fly in much more benign aircraft. They had gentle stall characteristics and were relatively safe. I was confident and flying was fun.

The aircraft I sit in now is nothing like those earlier planes. She has long, beautiful, shiny fiberglass wings and little winglets on the end. She is a plane with a pedigree, and she sparkles in the sunlight, flexing her wings in the breeze as if eager to fly. She was custom-built for a well-known pilot to fly in a world competition and has been winning all sorts of contests ever since. Most of the men at the airfield would love to have this plane.

The knot in my stomach is now the size of a bowling ball. If I had eaten anything, it would be splattered across the tarmac. Doubt seizes me. I am so scared. I want to turn and just run away.

Alongside the runway, a gaggle of male pilots huddle together, gossiping. Their eyes follow me into the cockpit, watching every move, waiting for the launch to commence.

My thoughts sway from one extreme to the other. I want to fly. I love flying more than anything in the world. I feel so alive in the sky. The sky is a place of awe and wonder, and it permeates every part of my being. I have this incredible plane, and she is all mine.

But I don't know if I can fly this plane, much less land it. The voice of the old pilot reminds me of the risk and of my lack of experience: You are going to kill yourself in *that plane*.

The tow plane, a white Pawnee with red trim, centers itself easily on the runway, dragging a tow rope behind it. It waits for me.

I close the canopy and give the thumbs up—the self-assured signal to launch—as if I mean it. I waggle my rudder, signaling the tow plane to go.

Alongside the runway the flock of male pilots gather, arms folded, standing in a cluster, following my launch. The Navy test pilot mutters something and they all laugh.

They take in every detail of my takeoff as I struggle to keep fifty feet of wingspan level until the wing has the speed to fly on its own. I veer off to the left and try desperately to bring the plane back to the center of the runway. I am awkward and uncoordinated, and I know this looks absolutely awful. And if I don't get this plane settled down, it could be dangerous, as well.

Along the sidelines, all eyes are on me.

This club attracts all sorts of members, from professional pilots to international financiers, to war-hardened vets and everyone in between. Aviation is a male domain, and soaring is a racing sport for this competitive crowd. The Navy test pilot says it's the best thing you can do with your clothes on. Some of the men clustered along the runway, watching my launch, will compete for a place on the U.S. World Team to compete in cross-country speed tasks that span hundreds of miles.

My plane's name is *Whiskey Oscar*. I'll tell you why I named her that later. Whiskey Oscar would come to teach me more than I could ever convey. But on this first flight, we have yet to become friends, much less student and mentor. She is an unknown beast, renowned for her speed, and she simply terrifies me.

I somehow follow the tow plane into the air, carefully balancing the plane from her CG (center of gravity) hook. This is where the tow rope connects to the belly of the aircraft. I've never flown a plane with a CG hook. There is no directional stability, unlike the sailplanes I've flown before, which are pulled aloft by a hook in their nose section. From the very first second, I must actively fly Whiskey Oscar, this plane I don't yet know how to fly, in formation, in sync with the actions of the tow pilot.

We rise into the air. I take a high tow to give myself time to get the feel of this plane. There is a haze around five thousand feet, and I separate from the Pawnee, who dives back to the Earth. Whiskey Oscar and I are alone in the sky.

The air is silent except for the pounding of my heart. No wind, no noise, no sensation of speed. Just the feel of the air under me, over me, surrounding me. Just the feel of these strange controls. Just the feel of movement as the plane banks and turns, carrying me with her. It is effortless to stay aloft. I have entered an alternative universe.

Whiskey Oscar's wings flex, as if in joy to finally be in the air. On the ground she is heavy and awkward, but here she is transformed into a graceful creature utterly, unabashedly in her element.

And I am flying her!

I am in love with this new airplane I barely know. I soar, cloud base above me, fields and orchards below. Time is irrelevant and it passes without my notice.

In the blink of an eye, over an hour has passed. I've lost no altitude. I could spend all day in the air in this endless dance with Whiskey Oscar, but this first flight is a familiarization flight. It is time I think about landing.

Landing. I have retractable gear (which way was down?); six flap settings ranging from negative eleven degrees to fifty-five degrees, and fifty feet of wing to contend with. What if a crosswind has picked up? What if there is sheer through the trees, that mix of unexpected, unstable air that can cause a sudden stall?

I look at the landing checklist which says UFSTALL: undercarriage, flaps, speed, trim, altitude, look out, land. One of the pilots at the airfield adds an extra F to his checklist; "You F*#!g Stall and You Die." It gets your attention. I add it to mine, too.

I crack my dive brakes to bleed off altitude. It takes time. This plane really flies, only, at the moment, I am too inexperienced to know that. I just know it's time to land.

"Don't let the airspeed get away from you," I had been warned.

Procedures help me focus. Undercarriage, down. Flaps, set. Speed . . . stay on top of the speed. Don't let it get away from you.

My checklist continues. Trim. Altitude, no traffic in the pattern. Looking, looking. No wind. Thank God there is no wind.

You f*#!g stall and you die.

God grant me the grace of children and idiots. I am obviously the latter.

This is it. I am in the pattern. There are no second chances. I descend; down, down, down. I don't see the trees reaching towards the belly of the aircraft. I do not see the grass. I barely see through my own inexperience and fear. Whiskey Oscar and I skim over the runway, waiting for her speed to dissipate. We finally settle. I open the air brakes, removing the lift from her wings, so she cannot even think about flying again. We roll to a stop. Our first flight is over.

I open the canopy and smell the springtime grass. I greedily inhale the fresh air. I think I've been holding my breath through the entire landing. Then a great big smile breaks across my face and I laugh. All the hope, the fear, and the joy of my first flight pour out of me. I am flooded with a range of emotions I cannot name or understand.

Whiskey Oscar would become my mentor, my muse, and my partner in adventure. She opened the door to a new language, one of heart, of inspiration, and of soul. She would teach me to connect with the Earth in awe as I soared down the spines of mountain ranges; she would show me the power of nature in a way I never imagined; and most of all she would force me to connect with myself.

Thanks to Whiskey Oscar and my own love of travel, I've come to see life as a road trip. Sometimes there are potholes, sometimes it's smooth sailing. Sometimes there are signs, sometimes not. Finding one's way can be challenging.

Life doesn't offer us a road map, but it does offer experience. And from our experiences might come wisdom. But wisdom is understood only in retrospect, and only if you are willing to confront life outside your comfort zone and contemplate the lessons that come with it. The lessons lie not in the adventure per se, but in your mindset, heart, and soul.

Come meet my guests as they share their bumps in the road and their extraordinary travels. From high altitude mountaineering to parenting, the people of this book are thoughtful and wise. They will raise your spirits, challenge your mindset, and send you on your own quest to create your very best life.

THE STORIES

CHAPTER ONE

A Question of Identity

"I would rather be real and be rejected than be fake and accepted."

–DARRYLL STINSON

We often define ourselves through our relationships, institutions, and material belongings. I went to this school; I have this degree; my child is this or that. Perhaps our identity rests upon what we drive, where we live, or what we wear.

This chapter is about the fragility of identity. It's about the power of rejection and the need for approval. It explores the consequences of following a path that is guided by external influences. Most of all, it's about the importance of learning to listen to your inner wisdom and building yourself from the inside out, rather than from the outside in.

My own story starts in New York in 1979. Events that unfolded would, over the next decade, would tear me down, build me up, and challenge my every assumption about the world around me.

New York, NY, 1979

I started a traditional and promising career path. Just where it would lead, I wasn't sure, but I eagerly joined the cadre of young graduates looking to make their way in the big, boisterous Big Apple.

New York is a cacophony of sound and energy, inequity, and possibility. Crowds bustle along teeming sidewalks, each person absorbed in their own world. Somehow, the mass of moving people possesses a sense of direction, and the sea of humanity flows along its way.

My father went to Wharton and so did I. After graduating in the midst of a recession, I was fortunate to get a job. I wanted to get involved with commodities or currency trading, but in those days, most New York financial circles were closed to women.

I found myself working in the corporate direct placement market. We structured deals in excess of $250 million (that was real money back in those days), funded leveraged buyouts, and had a front-row seat when interest rates hit 20 percent. It was a time of enormous transition. Variable rate mortgages were introduced for the first time and all the models for evaluating risk had to be re-created as the economy plunged into a rapidly accelerating interest rate environment the likes of which no one had ever experienced before.

I had a front-row seat to the unfolding financial saga of the times. I read about deals I was working on in the *Wall Street Journal*. I played squash at private clubs. I got engaged and married.

Overall, life looked good. But something was clearly wrong. I was having trouble swallowing. In my office one day, I found myself furtively digging my lunch out of my mouth to avoid choking. I was deeply exhausted. My limbs felt heavy, and my vision blurred. I wrote it off to the insanity of ninety-hour work weeks and constant stress.

I'd eventually be diagnosed with myasthenia gravis, a rare neurologic and autoimmune disease that causes muscle weakness. Little things like the ability to talk or walk, to swallow, read, and even to breathe became uncertain. With myasthenia, only about a third of the people recover to some degree, about a third spend their lives disabled, and about a third die.

My world, my life, my identity was suddenly teetering on an abyss that I simply couldn't comprehend. Nothing could have prepared me for what was to follow.

Part of the treatment for myasthenia is the removal of the thymus, a gland beneath the breastbone in your chest. Sometimes it can be removed with a smaller lateral incision near the clavicle. No such luck for me.

Surgery resulted in a long red scar right down the middle of my chest where my sternum was opened. I remember drawing a similar scar on all the models in magazines and catalogues with a bright red felt pen. When I was done defacing one catalogue, I'd move onto the next. Inside I was lost; stuck in a cloud of disbelief. What was I supposed to do? I had no roadmap for this.

I was suddenly on a plethora of drugs; some to combat muscle weakness, others to counteract the side effects of the original therapies. I didn't know if I would survive, and if I did, I had no idea what life might be like.

That experience challenged my identity on every level. I used to be strong; now I was weak. I used to be part of the world; now I was not. I used to be funny; now humor eluded me. The world went on and I was not a part of it.

My disability was an invisible one. Most people wouldn't notice the droop of my eyes or my labored gait. I put on my best public face and managed the unpredictability of my body and the impossibility of my drug regime in silence and solitude. I struggled with the simplest of tasks and I did my best to make it all look easy.

The dislocation I experienced with my previous life was stunning. Who was I in this no man's land of disability? What did my future hold? Would I even survive?

The reaction of people around me was to advise: "You shouldn't do this. Do you really want to do that? Maybe you should just rest."

The seemingly caring words boxed me in in every direction.

During this period, the surgeon who had operated on me asked if I'd be willing to speak to another young woman with myasthenia gravis. Her name was Debbie. She was a bit older than me, and much, much sicker. I had such feelings of despair and guilt whenever we got together. Was this where I was heading? It was not pretty. Debbie could barely speak in a croaking voice, and everyone told her she was crazy. She had to tape her eyelids open. She was weak and bedridden most of the time.

I, on the other hand, was doing well under the circumstances. I knew that one day of activity meant two days in bed. My ability to swallow had improved immensely, although I still muddled my words and was plagued with some double vision. Whenever Debbie and I got together, I felt such deep guilt because I was doing so much better than she was.

As time went on, my disease stabilized but the uncertainty remained. I did not know how I would feel on a particular day. I did not know if I could commit to a task. Without any direction or purpose, I was just digging a pit of worthlessness and despair that deepened with every year. Disability dominated my life despite my best efforts to rid myself of its constraints.

This experience turned my world upside down. It provided a brutal reality check on the degrees, networks, and possessions that so often define our paths and the expectations that mold our identities. They're all part of society's linear progression. Go to the right school, get the right job, marry the right person.

But what is the right school, the right job, or the right person? What happens when an unexpected detour derails your reality and what was right becomes wrong?

Just ask my guest Darryll Stinson.

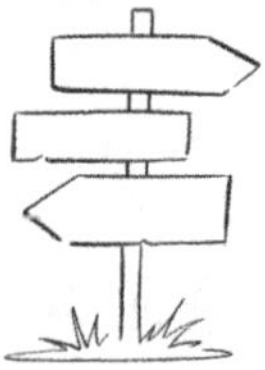

Meet My Guest, Darryll Stinson: Speaker, Coach, Pastor

I have to say that I smile just thinking of Darryll. He is an amazing man with an amazing story whose honesty and authenticity will touch your soul.

Darryll is an ex-athlete, entrepreneur, pastor, speaker, and a suicide survivor. As a child, he was intellectually gifted. He was one of two Black children in an advanced class, and as a gregarious, kind, and fun fellow, he was well liked by everyone who met him.

That is, until a group of students shamed him for his academically-oriented accomplishments. At that point, his life started to unravel as he sought the acceptance of his peers.

I literally changed everything I
was to fit into that community.

Darryll spent years trying to find his way back to his true self. And when he did, he realized that:

I would rather be real and rejected
than be fake and accepted.

Darryll's story will move you, motivate you, and have you rooting for him every step of the way.

Darryll Stinson: The Conversation

This conversation has been edited, but there's so much more to the story! When you have time, scan the QR code and you can listen to the original unedited conversation and view videos and photos of each guest. Or just visit BumpInTheRoad.us/Readers-Portal/ and sign in.

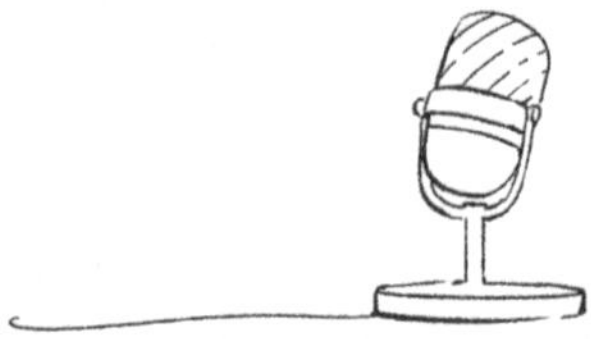

Darryll: My name is Darryll Stinson. I'm a speaker and a coach. I also have an organization called Second Chance Athletes, where we give athletes a second chance to succeed in life without the demands of sports.

I was a very smart, intellectual kid. My mother noticed that I was very gifted, so she put me in accelerated learning classes. What that meant for me was that I was one of two Black students in an all-white class, which wasn't a problem. They loved me. I was one of the smartest kids in the class. They cheated off of my tests.

They called me "goon." I was like this big, goofy, goony guy and I loved it. And I thought that since they loved me, everyone in the school must love me. Like, who didn't like Darryll?

One day I was on my way back from a bathroom break and I had this little wooden bathroom pass. I saw a group of Black students circle together and they were just cracking up, like having a great time. And I was like, man, let me get in on the jokes. I wanted to see what was so funny.

So, I walked over to them and I said, "Hey, y'all, what's so funny?"

No one answered.

I knew they heard me, so I spoke up a little louder and I said, "What y'all over there laughing about?"

And just as soon as I finished that sentence, someone turned towards me and said, "You are what's funny white boy. And I said white boy."

They all erupted in laughter. I walked away feeling rejected. I went around asking people, why did they call me white boy? I found out that I was known in our school as the Black kid who "talks and acts white."

That was the first time that I felt that sting of rejection and felt like who I was authentically wasn't enough to be liked or loved by others.

But what I've learned is that rejection affects all of us.

For some, it may be that you didn't get invited to drinks with your coworkers. For others, it may be a parent that never came around. For other people, it may be a promotion you never received at work.

Rejection has a way of making us feel like we're not good enough and that we don't matter.

I carried the seeds of rejection into the rest of my childhood, and I had this desire to fit in with this Black community.

Fast forward to me going into the seventh grade. My auntie and my first cousin's mother got shot and killed in broad daylight. My cousin's name is Chaz. Chaz and his mother lived in the projects. I was from the hood.

The difference is that I had drugs going on in my neighborhood. He had drugs going on in his house. I had violence going on in my community. He had it on his front porch.

Chaz's world was a much rougher environment than mine. And because Chaz's father was in prison and my dad and him were close, we decided to take Chaz in.

Chaz in the seventh grade had everything I wanted in the Black community. He had popularity, street cred, and esteem, and so he brought in this group of friends around me. At the age of, whatever age you are in seventh grade, they were already skipping school, trying to have sex, getting into fights, carrying around guns, and doing drugs.

They were living a whole different lifestyle than this kid who was still an all-A student with perfect attendance. Whenever we would hang out, they would make fun of me and it started to play on that insecurity that I had.

So, I literally changed everything I was to fit in with that community.

I changed the way that I talked, I changed the way that I walked, I changed the music I listened to. I even changed the way that I laughed. And it worked. They embraced me.

I got street cred. They called me a different type of goon. It was "street goon" this time and not "goofy goon."

And deep down inside I knew it
wasn't me who they accepted.
It was who I was pretending to be.

And as it was with me, I learned it is the same with a lot of people, because we all have this true, great desire to be liked and loved by other people.

We oftentimes go outside of our
character in order to be accepted.

The problem with that is that people can accept the fake you while the real you still feels rejected. If they knew who you really were, what you really believed, or what you really thought, you might not be included in the in crowd.

It's being able to separate the moment of rejection
from your identity, your worth, and your value.

What I have since learned about those students in the third grade is that they were projecting their fears and insecurities onto me in the form of mockery and jokes. So rather than deal with their own brokenness, they wanted me to feel bad about my authenticity.

None of them had the freedom or the courage to be themselves.

They were all fitting in, making poor decisions, scared to do anything that the clique wouldn't think was acceptable. And I was just naive enough to be myself and didn't understand the concept of projection.

Pat: How did you regain your authenticity after going that direction?

Darryll: I didn't.

I completely sold out.

I kept it up through college, and it wasn't until I had a career-ending back injury that took my path of being an NFL athlete away from me that I was forced to deal with this lack of identity.

I could no longer hide behind the street ego because I was battling an addiction to opioids. I could no longer hide behind my athletic success because it was no longer possible. And I had to find a way to be me again.

I had been faking it for so long, I didn't know what my real laugh was. What was my real laugh? What music did I really like? And what did I select just to please others?

I hit rock bottom. I did not know how to communicate my emotions.

I thought that vulnerability was weakness. You weren't supposed to show weakness; that was what I was taught as a man and as an athlete. So, I imploded. I kept my feelings all to myself and I started turning to drugs to deal with them. Long story short, it led to a really bad addiction that caused me to become suicidal. And I attempted suicide multiple times until I ended up in a psychiatric care facility in Detroit, Michigan. And there, I went through a lot of inner healing and had a very pivotal moment that gave me hope. From that experience, I began the process of figuring out who I was and peeling off all these layers of what I was pretending to be.

And along the way, I had an epiphany.

I would rather be real and be rejected
than to be fake and be accepted.

Thoughts For You to Ponder

Imagine your best self. What are the values that make you who you are?

How does your life differ from this 'best self' list?

Think of the people you spend time the most time with. Do they share the values of your best self? Do they pull you up or keep you down?

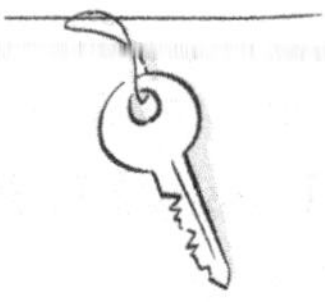

Key Takeaways

- Finding your most important inner values, and following them, is critical to navigating your life in a meaningful way
- Who you surround yourself with matters
- A meaningful and authentic life embraces vulnerability

CHAPTER TWO

Travel Abroad/Travel Within

"If it moves you, chase it."

–MARK PHILPOTT

What happens when you feel that things aren't quite right? Perhaps there's a nagging sensation, a dis-ease about life. A lack of meaning. It's not an intellectual knowing; it's a heartfelt knowing, and sometimes it takes a while for our mind to catch up to our heart and soul.

That unease often means that our innermost values are in conflict with our world. How do we reconnect with who we are? How do we separate our true selves from the beliefs and values instilled by our parents, our schools, and our society at large?

This gap between being true to yourself versus the persona you show to the world may create a crisis. Some call it a dark night of the soul. It's a place where your most cherished beliefs are stripped away and your deepest fears exposed. It's a place of black and white, do or die, where you must summon your courage and make the decision to move forward. It is an opportunity to rid yourself of your past demons to make room for new, unknown dreams.

For me, dreams were not a part of my disability landscape. I would vacillate between an intense yearning that went from life wish to death wish. It's not that I wanted to die, per se. I just passionately wanted to live. But before I could do that, I had to deal with disability, divorce, rejection, and isolation before I could learn to soar.

Connecticut 1983/Pennsylvania 1990

Coastal Connecticut is far removed from the bustle of New York. Long Island Sound laps lazily at the beach. Summer houses dot the shoreline and the gulls cry as they soar in the coastal breezes.

But the restful ambiance of Connecticut did nothing to stem the progression of my disease. After surgery, I found myself lost in a place with no landmarks. My very promising career was gone. I had no peer group. There was no internet, no way to connect with others. I had only a gaping abyss of uncertainty about my future, or if indeed there would even be one. I went from independent to dependent; from healthy to disabled; from directed to lost.

My first step was to decide to find happiness in the moment, even though the moment was nothing I had wished for or planned. I vividly remember coming to a four-way intersection of back-country roads in Connecticut, not too far from Long Island Sound. The street was lined with oaks that created a dappled shade on the road. The yellow center line was faded from the sun and from time. I could hear the sound of gulls and smell the scent of the sea.

At the intersection was a somewhat run-down white clapboard building with peeling green shutters. It just oozed old, aged New England. On the porch were magazine racks and a newspaper kiosk. It was a local store; the sort of market that sells everything from snacks to fishing worms.

I sat as if poised in time. My past was gone; my present uncertain. I did not know if I had a future. My so-called life was surrounded by obstacles, and here at this intersection was a four-way stop. That intersection seemed to define my life. Don't go here; don't do that. Stop, stop, stop.

I drew an imaginary line from stop sign to stop sign. In that box was safety, and I decided that I would find a way to cope with the impossible fatigue, health issues, and restrictions I faced.

As I drew that imaginary box, I knew deep down that I was ignoring essential parts of myself.

But I would find a way to be happy in my box.

My box closed in on me with each passing year. The boundaries were invisible and intangible, but they were very real. And they were unconsciously enforced by everyone around me.

But the choice to live in the box was mine. Soulful honesty and reflection weren't what I was looking for. I was looking to mold myself into this new limited life. I was looking to please the people around me; the people I depended on. But along the way, I totally forgot what pleased me.

Fast forward a little over a decade and a half, and my ex had run off with a new wife, a new job, and even a new dog. My myasthenia was thankfully stable, but my medication was becoming less and less reliable.

The problem was that titrating the drug dosage was impossible; too much medication had the same side effects as too little. I never knew if I was ahead or behind. It was like a funhouse mirror, where you are never quite sure what reflection is real and what is illusion. But in this not-so-fun-funhouse the implications of guessing incorrectly could be fatal.

Nevertheless, I decided to see what would happen if I cut back on my medications. I quietly reduced the doses and hoped for the best. I told no one about this. No doctor would take the risk. I balanced my health and energy carefully. I watched my body closely; sensitive to my mobility and breath. And careful observation was essential. I had started learning to fly.

Learning to fly was part life wish and part death wish. Given my reality on the ground, I didn't really care if I lived or died. I had lost everything that mattered to me: my family, my identity, my future. I didn't court death, but I wouldn't necessarily run from it, either.

On the life wish part of the equation, I found a boundless joy in flight. Flying was freedom, adventure, and a refusal to fit into a box. It was everything my soul craved.

But how could I get a flight physical under these circumstances? An answer appeared with the recommendation of a pathologist who did physicals on the side. All the pilots knew he was the go-to man for a less-than-rigorous exam.

His office was the morgue, deep in the subterranean corridors of the hospital. I entered a cavernous room with dull grey concrete slabs staged at regular intervals. The vent blew a cold draft across me, and a shiver ran through my body.

"Sit here," the doctor directed me to one of his lifeless slabs. I climbed up and crossed my arms, as if to ward off some spirit in the room. I was sitting on a dead man's table in pursuit of a life.

He listened to my heart and lungs through my shirt. "Any distinguishing scars?" he asked as he checked the various boxes on the medical form.

Admitting to a huge gash down the middle of my chest would have just opened a Pandora's Box of medical questions.

"None," I lied. I had to fly. It had become my raison d'etre. It was my bridge to sanity and some unrealized future. I needed this medical.

The doctor paused, as if to continue the conversation. I remember a friend telling me that the reason this guy did flight physicals was because he was lonely. He especially liked attractive young women.

I smiled my cutest smile and held my breath. I may have batted my eyelashes. Please, please just sign off on the friggin' paperwork, I thought.

His pen scratched across the paper. I breathed a deep sigh of relief. I was released to chase my dreams.

Meet My Guest, Mark Philpott: Corporate Executive, Traveler

Mark Philpott is a well-traveled corporate executive, entrepreneur, and adventurer. The twists and turns of his travels started off in Singapore. At the time, it appeared that Mark had it all. He was the consummate businessman, traveling the world, enjoying the highlife of great hotels, restaurants, and events. Until one day, depressed and alone in a hotel room, he realized this high-flying life was no longer working for him. And that insight led him on a profound quest that challenged his values and his very way of life.

Mark left his corporate job and spent two years traveling without a home, without possessions, sometimes sleeping on a park bench. He visited friends. He experienced the world from a very different perspective. And he emerged a very different man.

His travels started off being external: places, people, events. But in time his travels caused him to turn within, in search of his own truth. Reflecting on his life and travels to date from his sailboat in Australia where he now lives, Mark shares his story. His courage in searching for meaning and redefining his life is a lesson for all of us.

Mark Philpott: The Conversation

This conversation has been edited, but there's so much more to the story! When you have time, scan the QR code and you can listen to the original unedited conversation and view videos and photos of each guest. Or just visit BumpInTheRoad.us/Readers-Portal/ and sign in.

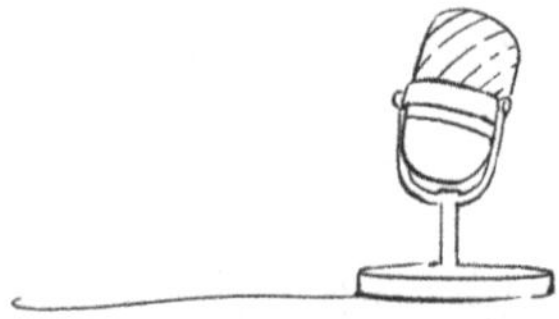

Mark: I was a corporate warrior for many years. I spent most of my life on aircraft traveling around the world for a big multinational company.

Before I knew it, a couple of decades had gone by, and I was getting older and perhaps none the wiser. I was living in Brussels in Belgium at the time. It was a very cold Sunday afternoon. I was depressed.

I was making shareholders of a company very rich and prosperous, but inside my soul, I was empty.

I was contemplating taking my own life.

The TV was on, and there was a story about a young sportsman who'd just had a horrific accident and became paralyzed. As I watched him, I thought, "There's somebody out there that's worse off than I am."

This young boy, who was in a wheelchair, was one of the best athletes in the world prior to his accident. And at the age of twenty-one, that dream was taken away from him in a freak accident.

I made the decision that I wanted to meet him. I don't really know why, but I just had a gut feeling that I should be doing this.

I reached out to him, and a few days later, I went to meet him. We eventually became good friends, and he helped me change my life. Because

I started to become compassionate for the first time in my life, thinking about somebody else, rather than about my own worries.

It taught me a big lesson, because I'd spent most of my life staying in fancy hotels, flying first class, and all those sorts of things. In my off time, I was able to go and watch Formula One Grand Prix and go to some expensive parties around the world.

And it was all very shallow.
This was the first time that reality hit me in the face.

It was a good wake up call for me. And it started me on a very lengthy journey.

It was through that experience that I ended up meeting Christopher Reeve, aka Superman. And that was another life-defining moment.

The lesson for me was that when we think of our own troubles as being life-shattering and life-ending, they often aren't, and there's always someone else out there that can teach us lessons.

Pat: One of the things you say is get out of your comfort zone. And I think once you're out of your comfort zone, that's the place where creativity can enter.

Mark: And also, authenticity.

I've spent some time as a homeless man.

And it was during that period of my life that I probably got to the closest form of my authenticity because I had stripped away everything else. There was no materialism; there was no business card or identity linked to a particular job or a big company.

I was out there in the wilderness of life. I look back at that period and it was a significant life-changing experience. It taught me a lot about myself, but also about the generosity of human beings if we open our eyes.

Pat: One of the things that you said was:

The journey to freedom was about not
doing what we're conditioned to do.

Mark: I remember sitting down with Christopher Reeve and Robin Williams. We talked about what's on the other side of the comfort zone. And Robin Williams said,

You know what's on the other side of your comfort zone?
It's the true you.

All I can say is that on the other side, if you give yourself the opportunity and if you let go of the fear, there is going to be something amazing that you can embrace and be part of.

Pat: What advice do you have for somebody facing their own bump in the road? If you could distill it down, what would you say to somebody?

Mark:

If it moves you, chase it.

You'll inevitably come across something in your life that just really pulls at your heartstrings. That's something worth chasing. See what you can make happen.

Thoughts For You to Ponder

Mark said, "The journey to freedom was about not doing what we're conditioned to do." Think about your daily routines. Can you name three things you are conditioned to do?

How do you feel about being without a set abode? Do you feel fear or freedom? Why?

Take some time this week and deliberately extend compassion to someone. Notice how that makes you feel.

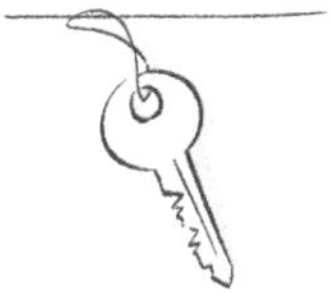

Key Takeaways

- The path forward is through your authentic self
- Develop compassion for others
- Find joy in daily life

CHAPTER THREE

Seeing The World Through a New Lens

"There are no rules."
-LIZ O'RIORDAN

We all belong to tribes that share our outlooks and passions. Perhaps you root for a certain sports team, or you belong to a club. Perhaps you're a lawyer, an engineer, or a doctor. Maybe you are part of a band. Our talents, hobbies, and interests naturally draw us into groups with others. And those groups can greatly influence how we see the world.

Our associations often define us. But they can also be temporary. Sometimes we're kicked out of a group; sometimes we leave voluntarily; sometimes we no longer qualify. What happens when, against our will, that identity is stripped away? How can we rebuild our reality and see ourselves from a new perspective?

This chapter explores how using a new lens to view one's world leads to new paradigms, both for me and for my guest Liz O'Riordan.

Pennsylvania 1990-1993

Illness redirected my life, then divorce destroyed it. Or so it seemed. I was unceremoniously kicked out of the family that had been my loving mainstay for a decade and a half. All the holidays and forays I'd shared with my beloved in-laws would go on without me.

Nothing seemed real. I was suddenly navigating life without all that I loved and valued. I was struggling on every level. Where could I go? What could I do? Why did no one care? That last question haunted me, resonating in my very soul, like a howl of pain that wouldn't go away.

In my quandary, I took a trip across the country, visiting friends and contemplating my future. A glider ride in Calistoga, CA (more on that later) introduced me to soaring. When I returned to Pennsylvania, I heard about a group of lawyers that flew on weekends. So, I invited myself out to the airport over a three-day weekend. Over those three days, something about soaring through the air with no engine touched my soul. Suddenly, I had a goal. I was going to learn to fly.

Given everything, this was a bit crazed. But I simply didn't care. I had to find something to live for, and this was something that touched my soul and fed my appetite for life.

The public thinks of soaring in a glider as a ride around an airport. But the sport of soaring involves navigating in a high-tech airplane without an engine on a cross-country task and hopefully returning to your original airport (this does not always happen). Without power, sailplanes depend on the energy in the sky.

Sometimes, lift is found in the wind bouncing off a ridge, or underneath a developing cloud. Sometimes air masses collide, and that instability creates an avenue of rising air. Sometimes it's a powerful force called wave that allows you to soar to thirty thousand feet or more.

Lift is a very real phenomenon, but it's also a metaphor. It's about being alert to your environment. It's about developing the skill to move forward and having the courage to leave your home airport behind.

I started flying with a World War II naval aviator at Kampel, a small, privately owned airfield on the western bank of the Susquehanna River.

The club had three gliders and a tow plane. The Blanik was a sturdy two-seat trainer. After soloing in that plane, I progressed to a 1-26, a low performance single seat plane. Think of it as graduating to your first sports car. It was a nimble, fun to fly plane that had a certain cult following in the aviation community.

Sam, my instructor, had one of the 1-26s weighed and balanced just for me. Without having to recalculate the weight distribution each time I flew and lug heavy weights in and out of the plane, I could show up at the airport and be airborne in short order. In my trusty 1-26 I was free to go as far as my imagination and the weather would allow. Sometimes I made it back to the airport; sometimes not. That wonderful little plane gave me unbounded freedom and joy.

But on one particular Saturday, a perfect Saturday with clouds popping in the sky and lift everywhere, I was without an airplane. "My" 1-26 had been committed to an airshow.

Every piece of my being wanted to be in the air more than anything in the world. And I was grounded. I was beyond pissed.

Flying had become more than a weekend hobby. It offered me the challenge and joy that had been so missing from my life for so long. Soaring, for me, was life itself. I had to find a way to get into the air on that perfect day.

I recalled hearing radio chatter from a group of pilots who told tales of racing through the sky and speeding down the Appalachian ridge, riding the energy of the air for hundreds of miles. Their base was an airport somewhere south.

So, in a fit of anger, I got in my car and decided to find them. I called ahead for directions. “Turn at the white barn,” I was told.

And, sure enough, an old white barn with ill-fitting siding appeared on my right. And shortly afterwards, an airport appeared, tucked into the countryside amidst the trees.

At the entrance I was greeted by a sign: Private Property. Do Not Enter. I drove past it.

Lining the runway were dozens of beautiful, sleek fiberglass ships ready for takeoff. Two tow planes staggered their efforts, launching the grid. This was pure magic! I had wandered into a club of “Sky Gods,” where world-class pilots scoffed at the laws of gravity to soar high through the sky for hours on end.

My heart leapt to my throat. I watched a series of takeoffs. I followed each plane into the air. I was one with their climb. This was a world of aviation beyond anything I’d ever experienced. I had to do this.

But the airplane situation there, I learned, wasn’t any better than it was at Kampel. To fly with this group, I needed my own airplane. So be it. I initiated a quest to find an airplane that would allow me to fly with this new tribe of “Sky Gods.” I had no idea what I’d set in motion when I left one airfield, and one tribe, for another.

Meet My Guest, Liz O'Riordan: Health Advocate, Surgeon

Liz O'Riordan had trained for decades to become a breast cancer surgeon in the United Kingdom Finally, settled into practice, she realized her childhood dream.

Each year, Liz treated thousands of women with breast cancer. But when she received her own diagnosis, she was stunned. Medical training didn't prepare her for the very human experience of being on the receiving end of medical care.

Liz faced surgery, radiation, and chemotherapy. Then, two years later, a recurrence led to still more treatment. As a result, Liz was no longer able to function as a surgeon.

Cancer had robbed me of the only thing
I ever wanted to do since I was a little girl.

With no hobbies, no social life, and no job, Liz faced a total redesign of her life.

How does one navigate a potentially life-threatening, career-destroying bump in the road and find some wisdom along the way? And what advice do you give to someone facing such a life-changing bump in the road?

"No rules," says Liz. And so much more.

Liz O'Riordan: The Conversation

This conversation has been edited, but there's so much more to the story! When you have time, scan the QR code and you can listen to the original unedited conversation and view videos and photos of each guest. Or just visit BumpInTheRoad.us/Readers-Portal/ and sign in.

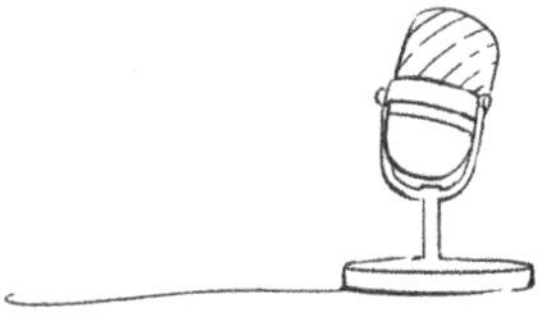

Liz: I was a consultant breast surgeon, and at the age of forty, I was diagnosed with stage three breast cancer myself. It was a huge shock because I knew too much.

I had treated patients with primary and secondary breast cancer, and suddenly I was about to go through every single treatment I gave my patients, and I knew everything. I knew my risk of recurrence. I knew what might happen to me. My husband and my parents knew nothing. And that power balance of knowledge was really, really hard.

I was treated by doctors and nurses I'd worked with, and they found it very hard to treat me. I had nine months of chemotherapy, a mastectomy, reconstruction, and radiotherapy. Three years after my diagnosis, my cancer came back locally on my chest wall, and that meant further surgery. I lost my reconstruction. It meant more radiotherapy because it grew in the same area. It meant having my ovaries out. And it also meant I had to retire as a surgeon, because the side effects of three operations in my armpit and the radiotherapy meant I couldn't move my shoulder properly.

Suddenly, at forty-five, cancer had robbed me of the only thing I ever wanted to do since I was a little girl.

Pat: Where did you go from there?

Liz: I don't know. I think it first hit me when my treatment had finished, and I had six months off to get my energy levels back.

And I just thought, who am I?

Because whenever I met people, I would inevitably say, "I'm a surgeon. I'm a doctor."

I defined myself by work and I'd spent twenty years of training through medical school and hospitals to be a surgeon.

I had wrongly stopped all the hobbies I used to do at school. I didn't have many friends. It was all job, exam, job, exam, write a paper, do a PhD, get the next job. I'd moved all the way across the country.

I had no social life. I'd lost my job. I was the most boring dinner party guest you could find. But I started to realize that work isn't everything. I started finding myself. I started reading and drawing and playing the piano again. And I found more friends and I started writing.

Writing for me was a massive outlet, because my experience wasn't real. I couldn't have cancer. I think I still haven't really had cancer unless I look in the mirror. My mind is protecting me, and writing was the way of getting it down on paper and dealing with it.

I started a blog. The blog led to me doing a TEDx talk. And that has now led to me speaking all over the world about a huge host of things from how to improve cancer care, to artificial intelligence, to telling children how to cope when things go wrong. I'm almost busier now that I've retired than I was as a consulting surgeon.

Pat: How are you enjoying the public speaking?

Liz: I love it. It's that theater. It's the buzz I used to get in an operating theater when I walked in. There's the nerves, and then you do an amazing operation and you think, wow, I nailed that.

I love getting in front of a crowd, but I work really, really hard. It probably takes about twenty or thirty hours to prepare each talk. And I do it from scratch every time. But to have a room full of people in your hand and make them laugh and make them cry and know they're going to take away your messages . . . Oh, it's like a drug.

Pat: You talked about the power imbalance as you were going through treatment. But there was another piece of that maybe you hadn't seen before. And that was the more emotional aspect and the personal aspect of going through cancer treatment. I don't think any of us are prepared for that.

Liz: You are so right.

As a doctor, cancer was normal.

It was mundane. I would see ten to twelve women a week with breast cancer. I would operate on them. And some of them would get passed on to the oncologist for chemo, or I would see them in a year's time.

I didn't get how bad it was.

And I think as a doctor, you must distance yourself because you can't cry every time, you'll just destroy yourself. So, it just becomes normal.

When it was my turn to sit, squeezing my husband's hand, staring at the floor, waiting to go in to find out if I had bad news, I suddenly got it. No one is lucky to catch cancer early enough because it hasn't spread. It's still cancer. And that whole emotional rollercoaster of "Am I going to die? In two years' time, will I still be alive? Can I plan? How do I get over never having children?" There's also the guilt you feel at bringing that into a relationship and how menopause affects your marriage! I had no idea.

It's not just an operation and a word.

Pat: I've always thought cancer has a potential to be a portal into a more conscious life. I think that you discover the value of time and the beauty of the day. And that seems to be something that runs through many people's cancer experiences.

Liz: It's the same for me.

I suddenly realized that what was important in life was friends and family and making memories.

I didn't want to be remembered for being a surgeon, I wanted to be remembered for all the joy I brought to other people. It's about making friends, it's about traveling. It's about making new memories. And you realize that you don't need half the things you have. That's what's important.

Pat: I totally agree. I can certainly say for me, it's been a shift away from materialism. All I need is my computer, maybe my microphone, and my cameras, and I'm a perfectly happy camper.

Liz: I still like a nice pair of shoes every now and then!

Pat: Of all the changes you've encountered, and you've been through a lot, what do you take away from it? What is the deepest change that you see in your life?

Liz: I think it's realizing that:

Life isn't a straight line.

Life throws you curve balls, and you need those curve balls to help you learn and grow along the way.

It's okay if things don't work out, maybe they didn't work out for a reason.

I think when you have a defined career, like medicine, you are told this is it, there is only one way to go, do not pass, go. And I think that's wrong. We need to send people out to explore the huge variety of life.

Pat: We're both pretty active on social media. I have a travel contingent, and I have a cancer contingent. It's kind of an odd combination. But my favorite contingent is the cancer contingent. I enjoy the people because they're heartfelt, as they deal with deep issues. They have something to say that I think has wisdom for all of us.

Liz: I think you're right. I had no idea the cancer community existed before I was diagnosed. It is a whole new world and there's the good, the bad, and the ugly. And there are times when it just gives me the lift and the support I need. I don't know how I would have coped if it wasn't for cancer patients on social media, because I didn't see another cancer patient physically during my treatment. I had no one else to talk to. All my support was online.

Pat: Online was just getting going when I was diagnosed. That was back in 2009. I thought I would hate social media. I did it to build a website and now I am hooked. I meet the best people from all over the world through social media. It's just amazing.

And I think in the cancer community, it's been pivotal for so many people. It's been a place for people to find connections and to find advice.

Liz: It's amazing. You can follow scientific conferences and you can ask doctors. I think we're all equal on the internet. Instead of being a nervous patient with a list of questions you're too embarrassed to ask your doctor, on Twitter you can be brave. You can be confident. You can just ask someone. You've got nothing to lose. Same on Facebook and Instagram. I think that's a great way of redressing that power balance.

Pat: There is a power disbalance in medicine. You've seen it from both sides.

Liz: When I was first training, I used to have women who would come to me with inches of papers of trials they'd printed off the internet. And I'd think, oh my God, it's a difficult patient. They've got all these trials I haven't heard of. And I was meant to be the expert and I hated it. Then I was the patient, and suddenly I was the one researching the trials. I felt so awkward emailing my doctor saying, could you have a look at this, as if to suggest that I might know more than her.

As a doctor, you don't realize that every single patient's life is really important to them. And they don't realize you are not investing all your time into helping them.

A patient is just one of 200, 300, 400 you may treat a year. But when you are a patient, you are the most important cancer patient in your doctor's job. Does that make sense?

Pat: It makes total sense. I saw my doctors as working for me to assist me with where I wanted to go. I was intent on getting into a clinical trial at Stanford and I told my oncologist. I wanted him to open the door, which he willingly did, but I was the one who did all the research and found the clinical trial. But the most interesting thing to come out of my pushing for this trial was that I found out they had misdiagnosed my cancer. I say to everybody: Do what you need to do, research it, but take charge because it is your life, and nobody is as invested as you are.

Liz: And your doctor may not like it, but they're not the one who's living with it.

I had no idea what it was like to live with a cancer diagnosis. I thought I knew everything because I treated women.

I saw them all the time. But until you are living with that bombshell of how it affects every single aspect of your life, you can't understand it.

Pat: No. And our society focuses on diagnosis and treatment, sometimes very effectively. But no one addresses the post-treatment phase, which is the rest of your life. It has profound psychological and spiritual issues, and yet we don't address them. To some extent, we can't, because our institutions aren't set up them do this, but I think we can address it through the power of story. And I think that's where the wisdom lies in terms of trying to figure out this dance we do with mortality.

Liz: I think you're right. For me, the hardest part was after a year, when my surgeon said, "I'll see you in a year."

When you have chemo, you're seen regularly. All of a sudden, you wonder what happens next? How do I know if it's coming back? How do I cope with the side effects? How do I live? How do I cope with my husband, all of that? How do I live? How do I cope with my husband? You go into this whirlpool of despair.

And I think this is where stories have such value. They explain that this is what it's like a year after diagnosis. This is what is like three years after the end of treatment. When you first have a recurrence, this is what it's like, and this is what you do.

But the patient must be ready to hear that information, because you don't want to hear about recurrence a day after your diagnosis. When the surgeon is giving you good news, saying it's all gone, they can't say oh, by the way, it might come back and kill you. It's very hard as a doctor to know when to tell patients that.

For me, it was the guilt I felt when someone's cancer came back. I almost wanted to have it because I didn't want them to have it. And there's a sense of wanting your cancer to come back so you can stop waiting for it to happen and move on.

But you obviously don't want it to come back. It's just so irrational.

Pat: It is irrational. I think we get this idea implanted in our minds that it's inevitable, it will come back. So, you live in this very strange stress point of, am I living, am I dying? What's going on? What's going to happen?

Liz: I used to worry about the numbers; what was my risk of recurrence? I realized I may have a 40 percent chance of being alive in ten years, but I don't know whether I'm the 40 percent or the 60 percent. And for me, the chance of my cancer coming back is fifty/fifty. It happens or it doesn't. And I can do everything. I can eat well, I can exercise, and it may still come back.

I don't have any control.

Realizing that really, really helped me. I just live my life now. I make plans, and if something happens, I deal with it, but I can't put my life on hold.

Pat: There's a question I'd love to ask. If you could rewrite your story, would you, and how would you rewrite it?

Liz: That's really interesting. I guess you're saying, would I rewrite the cancer diagnosis? I honestly don't think I would.

I'm a better person for having cancer. I am more fulfilled. I found an inner strength I never knew I had. I've got a massive friendship circle. I've developed a new zest for life.

Before I got cancer, I was a surgeon doing long hours. It was all about the patients. It was me and my husband and very little outside. And I thought that would be my life until I was sixty. And although it was horrific having cancer, and I wouldn't want it again, the positives that have come from it outweigh the negatives. Isn't that crazy?

Pat: No, I don't think it is. I think that many people who face a bump in the road either hit a point of transformation or they don't. And transformation is hard. It's really difficult, but the positive things that can come out of choosing to take that path are just astonishing. You'll go places you would never have expected, and you never could have anticipated. And maybe that's a good life lesson in that we should let go of some of our expectations and just see where life takes us.

Liz: So, I haven't shared this with many people, the day before my mastectomy, I was about to lose my breast. We live near some farmer's fields, and my husband and I walked through them. I stripped off topless in the middle of a cornfield and he took a photo. I would never do that before. And I've never shown it to anyone, but just that kind of feeling of:

You can do anything within reason and
just let go and see who you really are.

Pat: What advice would you give to somebody facing their own bump in the road?

Liz: I would say there are no rules.

Thoughts For You to Ponder

Have you ever had to give up something you loved?

How did you feel about the loss?

What did you ultimately gain?

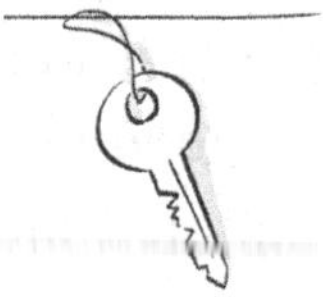

Key Takeaways

- Life isn't a straight line
- There is life after loss
- There are no predetermined rules in finding your path in life

CHAPTER FOUR

Dare to Explore: A Global Road Trip

"Not one single leg of my journey was ever the exact route that I had planned."

–ANGELA MAXWELL

The metaphor of the road trip is an old one, embedded in our discourse. Fork in the road; bump in the road; the road to ruin. Twists and turns. What is the magic of the road?

We travel, we meet people, and we see new things. We come back with stories to tell and somehow the best stories aren't just about a trip, but about how travel has changed us.

This chapter is about how my guest and I both experience an indefinable bit of dis-ease that leads to an unplanned, life changing road trip. What are we searching for? What do we find? Where will it lead?

Read on.

Road Trip: Pennsylvania to California and Back 1995-1996

It was winter, and East Coast winters are not amenable to flying. The grey overcast skies mean no lift. The damp cold permeates everything, and all the planes get tucked safely away in their hangars, in the dark, waiting, like the pilots, for spring.

I passed the sign at the entrance to the airfield that says "Private Property. No Trespassing," and drove down to the main hangar where I parked my car. There is a control tower that sits atop the airport office. It was in a state of disrepair, its entry locked.

I yanked open the door to the main office, the one that sticks in its frame. A group of pilots were sprawled on the ragged furniture in front of a TV, watching a football game, hooting and hollering, and drinking beer. The beer came from the green refrigerator out in the hangar, which had a hole punched conveniently into the door, allowing the tap to protrude. There was no need to even open the door.

Weekend after weekend, the winter weather closed in. I distracted myself by exploring the dozens of old antique stores scattered throughout the Pennsylvania countryside. I alternated my weekends between browsing cold, drafty barns stuffed with old artifacts, with hanging out at the airfield stuffed with grumpy, rumpled pilots. In one place I drank in history, in the other I drank in beer. Winter lasted forever.

After my divorce, workwise, I had no current skills. I fell back on my finance days and took the Series 7 securities exam and went to work as an investment advisor. After navigating an international theatre of billions of dollars of acquisitions and divestitures, stock offerings, and other cool and creative stuff in the world of finance, I was bored out of my mind with giving investment advice to a bunch of arrogant surgeons.

I looked at each client as X number of dollars when they walked in the door. And nearly all of my clients were surgeons, as was my ex, so I did derive a bit of perverse pleasure from that. Had I been able to reframe my circumstances as an opportunity to genuinely help others, I was sitting on an enviable and affluent network from which to build a block of business. But I couldn't make that leap. I was still consumed by anger over my divorce and perceived abandonment.

You will not be punished for your anger;
you will be punished by your anger.
–Buddha

I was displaced, in an untenable void between earthbound anger and skyward bliss. My life felt like one of those Mardi Gras masks, where one face is smiling and the other is crying. That fracture between my life in the air and on the ground was becoming more and more difficult to navigate; particularly during those long winter months.

While the romance of flying never faded, the reality of life at the airfield had. I did not see myself continuing in this pattern of persevering through the grey of winter year after year. A case of pneumonia forced me to take some time off and confront my life. I was living in a place I never wanted to live. I hated my house. I hated this part of the country. I hated my job.

This was not my life.

It was at that moment that I decided to take the summer off with Whiskey Oscar on a cross-country adventure.

This was the mid-1990s. Smart phones didn't exist. There were no websites, no Google, not much of anything that would help with some trip planning. As a result, my plans were somewhat nebulous. That summer, I headed west, uncertain about my destination other than the dim recognition that I needed one.

My first destination was Oshkosh, Wisconsin for an annual gathering of aviation enthusiasts. It's seven straight days of aerobatics, history, and camaraderie. For one week, this obscure little airport becomes the busiest airport in the world. And Whiskey Oscar and I were in the show.

Oshkosh rocked. I found inspiration in the stories of the WASPs, the women pilots from World War II who had put their lives on the line and went unrecognized for decades. I bought a Fiffinella pin, the WASP mascot designed by Walt Disney, and mounted it in my cockpit. I flew an ultralight with pontoons from the seaplane base. I told the pilot about my summer quest. "You're going in search of your soul," he responded.

While I thought I had found my soul in the sky, I had yet to find it on terra firma. That summer, I soared the Rockies, the Sierra, and places in between. I traveled from California wine country to Canada, down to Santa Fe, then back east.

The entire aviation-themed trip was one surprise after another. I "discovered" the Badlands in South Dakota and went flying with a helicopter crew. I soared the ridges above Aspen. I viewed Utah and all its splendor from high above. And In South Dakota, I met a little girl who asked me what was in the long, sleek trailer attached to my car. "A sailplane," I responded, and I opened the trailer so she could see inside.

The fuselage was carefully cradled in the center, with the beautiful, fiberglass wings safely stowed on either side.

The little girl's eyes opened wide. "Does she have a name?" she asked.

"Whiskey Oscar," I responded.

Planes and pilots are called by their contest letters and numbers, which are plastered on the tail in large letters. In the air, I would hear Tango One calling good naturedly on the radio, "Whiskey Oscar, passing you on the left." A few minutes later his voice would reappear, "Whiskey Oscar, passing you on the right."

Learning to fly fast was a slow task, at least for me.

In the air and sometimes on the ground, we knew each other by our contest letters. The problem with letters is that they lead to some interpretation. So, Hotel Hotel (HH) became Happy Hooker. Most of the men chose numbers for their contest IDs, since numbers didn't lend themselves to such creativity.

I was clueless about this naming convention. I wanted "Whiskey" to be one of my contest letters. Whiskey Sierra was unavailable, so I chose the letter "O" for Oscar. The choice wasn't premeditated any more than my flying career. So, she–we–became known as Whiskey Oscar (WO).

Over time, I came to associate this beautiful, graceful craft with a string of sayings, none of which I shared with anyone. Two that seemed to stick were "Women Only" and "Wild One."

Women Only was certainly suitable for my foray into this very male bastion of sport. I was the only woman flying a high-performance plane. I was the only female pilot at the picnic tables at night, sharing stories of the day's flight.

My other unknown moniker for Whiskey Oscar was Wild One. I didn't really think of myself that way, but when you consider that in just over a decade, I had gone from Wall Street, to disability, to flying this magnificent plane, and now taking her on a cross-country adventure, I had to pause. Perhaps it was a serendipitous choice of contest letters after all.

That summer, going cross-country with Whiskey Oscar, I didn't know if travel was the answer to my malaise, but the trip gave me the excuse to get out of Dodge, to get some distance from things, and to reconsider my life and what I wanted out of it. I really didn't have a clue.

Soaring was my lifeline. It gave me structure and adventure. It consumed me, which left little time to consider what might actually be missing from my life. In my case, the answer was me, but that wasn't something I was ready to understand. I just hoped that this trip might gently prod me in the right direction, whatever that might be.

Meet My Guest, Angela Maxwell: Adventurer, World Traveler

At thirty-two years old, Angela Maxwell had a wonderful life. But something was missing.

Often times we wait for some type of crisis to change things . . . I was doing really well . . . everything was actually quite good . . . but I felt like I was seeking something more.

A story about an inmate that walked the jail yard and walked the equivalent of an around the world trip intrigued her. Who else had done such a thing? Books by solo female adventurers such as Ffyona Campbell, Rosie Swale Pope, Robin Davidsons, and Jane Goodall fueled her imagination and wanderlust.

So, Angela decided to walk around the world. She left Bend, Oregon, on May 2, 2014.

I was a complete amateur. Just a few day hikes.

Her first stop after Oregon was Australia, where she hiked from south to north along the west coast.

Australia will always be my favorite country because it was the . . . harshest. It stripped me of the identity of who I was.

Yet for all its hardships, including sun blisters and heat stroke, Australia also provided Angela with the knowing that this could be done.

Six and a half years, fourteen countries, and eleven pairs of shoes later, Angela observed:

Courage is something that doesn't take a grand adventure . . . Wherever we meet the edges in our life . . . anything beyond our comfort is being courageous.

Angela Maxwell: The Conversation

This conversation has been edited, but there's so much more to the story! When you have time, scan the QR code and you can listen to the original unedited conversation and view videos and photos of each guest. Or just visit BumpInTheRoad.us/Readers-Portal/ and sign in.

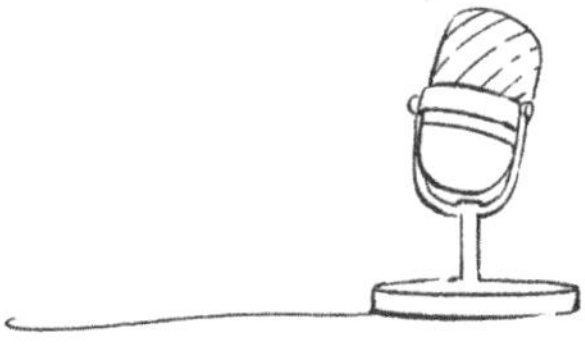

Angela: I'm Angela Maxwell, and on May 2, 2014, I left Bend, Oregon, to walk my way around the world. I walked across four continents, fourteen countries, and a handful of islands. It took six and a half years, and I went through about eleven pairs of shoes and lots of Cup O' Noodles and oatmeal. And I just finished on December 16th, 2020.

I started in Bend, Oregon, and walked to Portland, which took about two weeks. I had already planned that I would start in Australia. Of course, I was a complete amateur, just a few day hikes. I would take a little backpack with a sandwich and water and maybe go hiking for the day, maybe go camping, but the car was nearby and at least I knew in two days I could go home and take a shower.

First, I flew from Portland to Perth, which is in Southwest Australia. I walked north towards Darwin and I ended in a small Aboriginal community called Kalumburu.

I have a friend who described my trek of walking and flying well. She says that I've "waltzed around the world."

I walked across Australia, and then I went to Vietnam. I was planning to do Southeast Asia, but within ten days I had gotten dengue fever. I had to reevaluate what I wanted to do.

Vietnam was a culture shock to go from the outback to people and cars and humidity. And I realized while I was healing from dengue that I wanted to be back in solitude. So, I flew to Ulan Bator, Mongolia, and made my way through central Asia to Istanbul in Turkey. From there I decided to go do Scotland and England. And then I went back and did Sardinia and Sicily, the two Italian islands.

An adventure is really about where it takes us, who we meet, and the experiences along the way. And so, while I was waiting for the ability to get back into Europe due to visa considerations, I walked across New Zealand. Then I went back to finish parts of England and did the Northern parts of Europe, Holland, Belgium, and parts of France.

Pat: Any favorite spots?

Angela: Oh, yes. And it depends on the parameter.

Australia will always be my favorite country because it was the first continent. It was the harshest. It stripped me of the identity of who I was.

I was a thirty-two-year-old woman at the time. I had dirt in my fingernails. I hadn't showered in a month, and yet I felt so empowered, strong, and very beautiful, as dirty as I was. I loved the solitude. Australia gave me the foundation and the encouragement that if I could survive that and enjoy it, surely I could keep walking for years to come.

I think Australia was my favorite as a foundation, and Sardinia, the Italian island, was one of the most beautiful. And New Zealand, because there were no animals or venomous snakes to worry about! The scenery is gorgeous, and I like the lifestyle.

Pat: How much advanced planning and research did you do?

Angela: Not too much. I wanted this to be an intuitive mapping experience. For example, I'd say, "I'm going to do Perth to Darwin."

However, I didn't do Darwin. I ended in Kalumburu because of the people I met along the way.

Or from the trek from Tbilisi, Georgia to Istanbul. I could go central, or I could stay up north along the Black Sea. I would just start out and then let the journey shape itself. Not one single leg of my journey was ever the exact route that I had planned.

Pat: When you were getting ready to take off, was there a place of dis-ease, if you will; just discomfort with your current life? Was there an event that triggered this?

Angela: That's a great question. Not at all. I was doing phenomenally well. I had my own coaching and consulting business. It was remote. I could do it from anywhere. I had just moved to Bend a few months before. Got myself a little cottage right downtown. I could walk everywhere, and everything was actually quite settled. But I felt like I was still seeking something more.

I was in an art class, and I heard about a prisoner who had walked the equivalent of the distance around the world in the prison yard. That's where the light bulb went off, and I thought,

"That's a brilliant idea! Who has walked around the world? Surely someone's tried. Who's done it? What men have done it? Has a woman done it? Did they walk, did they cycle? What routes did they take?"

I just started devouring stories and getting inspired and encouraged. I wouldn't have made it through if it weren't for people who were sharing their stories. It helped me to get started.

Pat: Any particular heroes that really inspired you?

Angela: It's interesting. A lot of people jumped to Cheryl Strayed in *Wild*. I hadn't actually heard about her book. But there's Ffyona Campbell, who walked across four continents over a decade or so. And there's Rosewell Pope who, at fifty-seven, left her home in Wales to run solo around the world. There's also Rob Davidson, who took camels across Australia in the seventies.

And then there are the classics. There are accounts of what it was like for women like Jane Goodall. There are stories of women who have done things a little bit outside of the box. There are a tremendous number of female adventurers that most people never know of. And I had to really dig deep to find those women.

Pat: A travel adventure like that becomes an adventure inward, doesn't it?

Angela: I think that ultimately it kind of has to be. Even if someone doesn't have a foundational belief in spirit or religion or anything, they find themselves connecting to nature. There's a way of just getting in touch with your thoughts.

For me, it was very much a spiritual pilgrimage. I wanted the walk to take me on an adventure. I didn't want to shape my adventure. I wanted the walk to shape me.

I wanted to fine-tune my intuitive sense of where I'm going. And to continue that on in my life now.

My motto that I'm working with in my life today is:

You really never know what lies around the corner.

Pat: I totally agree. I've come to see life as a road trip.

Angela: Isn't it? Whether it's hiking the Pacific Crest Trail, or walking around the world, or motherhood, marriage, having a job, or wanting to contribute to the world, there are all these different paths and we're all taking them together in this parallel adventure.

Pat: How hard has it been to integrate back into so-called normal life and how do you hang on to that special spiritual connection that comes with a trip like the one you took?

Angela: When people ask me, "Who was the Angela who left Bend and who is the one who came back?" I can easily say, "I left still a bit of an adolescent. And through the walk, I feel like I've come back a little bit more mature in the sense that I'm comfortable in my skin and confident in making my own decisions."

I continue to tune myself to what I believe is guiding me.

It's about what feels right for me and not listening so much to the external as much as the internal.

Pat: What is courage to you?

Angela: I see courage as a choice. I called my TEDx talk "Courage is a Verb" because I see courage as motion. It is a choice we must step into. I think a lot of people have heard that when you're fearless, it's not that you won't be afraid, it's that you keep moving forward anyway.

When people ask, "Weren't you afraid being a woman alone, sleeping in a tent almost all the time in the bushes?"

I absolutely was every day. There was a daily moment of fear. Would I find a good camping spot that night? Was it going to be safe? Would I make it to this lake in time to fill up on water? There were always moments of fear and anxiety.

Courage is something that doesn't take a grand adventure.

It's wherever we meet the edges in our life. Anything beyond our comfort zone, to me, is being courageous.

I was alone in Mongolia, in a ravine, having had the most terrifying experience in my life (Angela was raped while in her tent in Mongolia), waiting for the sun to rise and then saying, "Okay, I'm at this pivotal point, do I give up and go home? I mean, I don't even have a home, but do I just go back to the normal status quo or do I find this innate strength and courage?"

I believe we all have to keep walking,
and it's going to be terrifying.

And anything outside of our comfort zone is a risk.

If I had never walked around the world, would I have ever really known what it feels like to choose courage? I believe I'm a better human being by deciding to follow my heart.

I can't tell you how many people say, "Oh, you are so brave."

I'm not that brave. But the thing is that we all have the innate ability to be brave. We all have an innate ability to love; to have compassion and empathy for people. We all have the ability to choose courage.

I think it can be overlooked that:

It takes a choice of courage to go within yourself.

It is courageous to see your blind spots; to let other people also see your true vulnerability and to let them support you through that.

*To me, being vulnerable, being open and honest,
is the deepest sense of connection we can have.*

I think going within ourselves and really discovering what we think, what we feel, how we see the world, and how we see ourselves is an act of courage.

Pat: And it's interesting to look at our beliefs, isn't it? And to look at how they can be stripped away. And all of a sudden you realize what is true.

Angela: Yes.

I believe we have the ability to create our own belief systems.

What we choose to agree upon, and what we disagree with, is also what shapes our personality and how we engage with people, communities, and ultimately within the world.

Pat: There is a quote of yours that I really liked:

*Embracing curiosity and open-mindedness
is a powerful way to experience the Earth.*

Angela: The moment we think we know the magic of the universe, we stop being curious.

If we can stay open-minded and curious about what we're experiencing, it is like a whole other world. And I think that is what perpetuates more open-mindedness within ourselves and within the world. Ultimately, a lot of the problems I think we run into are from the lack of compassion and the ability to stay curious and open to what other people think and how they feel.

None of us want to live in a world with everyone feeling the same way about something. We forget that we actually appreciate the contrast of life. And to be open-minded to that is what creates deeper connections.

We're just humans and we all want the same things. We want to be loved. We want to love. We want to be happy and successful and healthy and safe.

Ultimately, I realized on the walk that borders definitely don't define us; that we're all the same.

Pat: I agree. I think these emotional and spiritual needs transcend any arbitrary definition of country, border, person, color, or anything else.

Angela: Absolutely. And that travel is what opens us up to those experiences.

Pat: When you're out there beyond your comfort zone, a friend of mine calls it "the void," there's all this possibility. There's no prescribed route. There's nothing you must do. There's not a time clock on you. What do you want to create? It's such a cool place to be.

Angela: Yeah. Oftentimes, the word unknown comes up.

I feel the most comfortable in the unknown.

It's scary for most people because we want to *know*. We want to know how things work. We love it when we have a defined future goal. But in the unknown, the magic of what could spontaneously show up in your life could take you in a different direction. Most people regret what they didn't do.

Pat: One of my favorite quotes from you is, "We will all at some point need to sacrifice comfort for the integrity of our heart."

Can you have both?

Angela: Absolutely. Before I left for the walk, comfort was being able to get pizza delivered to my door. Comfort was that I could turn on Netflix. I could just hit a button and my gas fireplace would turn on.

Now, comfort is knowing who I am. Comfort is that I know my strengths and weaknesses. I know the places where I can grow and expand as a person. I know those edges. And so, when we talked about anything beyond the comfort zone, my comfort zone is wider.

Pat: If you could distill this amazing adventure down to three or four points to leave with people, what would you tell them?

Angela: It's never too late to change. You are naturally born strong, courageous, beautiful, and perfect, and you can honestly do and be anything that you want. And I do believe that life itself is the greatest adventure we'll ever have.

Thoughts For You to Ponder

Can you recall a time in your life where you felt a vague dis-ease? What was that feeling trying to tell you?

Think of a time you stepped outside of your comfort zone. How did it make you feel? Did you feel fearful, curious, or perhaps courageous?

Embrace your curiosity for a week. Where did it take you?

Key Takeaways

- "Courage is something that doesn't take a grand adventure . . . Wherever we meet the edges in our life . . . anything beyond our comfort is being courageous"
- Broadening our experiences broadens our comfort zone
- Travel can become a spiritual pilgrimage as we look to learn about ourselves

CHAPTER FIVE

Daring to Dream

"The biggest thing I came away with was that I wanted to live more fully and follow my wildest dreams."

–CHRIS DAHL-BREDINE

We like to think we control our lives. We work hard, gain skills, and we progress. We attribute meaning to our efforts and goals.

But sometimes an event forces us to reconsider our world view. How much do we really control? And what is the implication of losing that control? What can we learn when we learn to let go?

That, and more, is in this chapter.

Minden, Nevada, 1999

Lake Tahoe was originally the terrain of nomadic Indian tribes until it was discovered by John C. Fremont in 1844. That discovery, along with the discovery of silver in nearby Virginia City, put the region on the map.

Just east of the lake, in the valley several thousand feet below, lies Minden, Nevada. The airport at Minden was built in 1942 as a military training base. Today, it is an international mecca for sailplane pilots. Celebrities, aviation enthusiasts, and even astronauts flock to this high desert airfield where strong thermals and mountain wave enable one to go far, go high, and go fast. Flying to thirty thousand feet or more on a good wave day is relatively easy. And long runs down the mountain ranges can take a very experienced (and daring) pilot hundreds of miles from Tahoe to the Mojave and back. Minden is aviation hog heaven for the motorless crowd.

Among those pilots were Donald Engen, Director of the Smithsonian's Air and Space Museum, and his longtime friend, Bill Ivans. Bill was the Honorary Vice President of the Soaring Society of America and a very experienced pilot with world speed records and over 7,500 hours of flying time.

This particular day in Minden was a good soaring day; sunny in the morning, although thunderstorms would later roll through the valley. The power of a storm is both good and bad. It indicates highly unstable air (which is good for soaring), but there can be downsides, too.

That day, Engen and Ivans were flying a massive, two-seat Nimbus 4DM sailplane; a plane that can glide at high speed for *hundreds* of miles. All this makes it the plane of choice for long, cross-country cruising and for setting distance records.

It was a typical morning in the high desert. The sky was clear, the air was warming, and thermals were starting to pop. Engen and Ivans were in the air, east of the airport. They banked the plane to catch some lift when suddenly the plane entered a spin. The stress caused the wings to rip away from the aircraft and they slammed into the ground at 200 mph.

The aviation community was stunned.

The National Transportation Safety Board (NTSB) report cited a combination of eyewitness accounts and manufacturer data, concluding that the spinning plane had exceeded the never exceed speed (Vne).

In less than ten seconds, it was all over.

A heavy heart hung over the airfield. Tom Stowers from High Country Soaring noted that this accident would have international ramifications. The mood was somber. People were in a state of depressed shock. If it could happen to those two experienced pilots, it could happen to anyone. Call it ego, call it denial, but the illusion of invincibility is a key ingredient of a cross-country pilot's psyche.

To this day, I still don't believe this happened to two such seasoned pilots. I too have spun out of a thermal when I was just learning to fly. I was in a steep bank, flying as slowly as possible to maximize the rate of climb. But I got too slow and one wing stalled, sending the plane into a spin. The plane rotated once, twice, then three times. I was mesmerized by the sight of the rotating Earth. It was so beautiful.

I came to my senses and righted the aircraft. My World War II naval aviator-instructor, Silent Sam (as I called him for his stunning lack of conversation), laughed in the back seat. We spent the rest of the day doing some spin training. It was actually great fun.

Different planes spin differently. Some are benign, some not. I remember the Navy test pilot telling me tales of spinning a plane like Whiskey Oscar.

"Ever spin a 20?" the naval test pilot asked, laughing. "Most frightening thing I've ever done."

He paused for effect.

"First it enters sorta slowly," he said in the drawl that all military pilots of a certain age seem to have, "and the first rotation's not too bad. But then it really *whips* around. Ya gotta be careful to have your flaps full negative, or you'll *rip* the wings off."

He flung his arms back dramatically to demonstrate the effect of wings stressed in a spin.

"Then ya go to recover, and it tucks." He paused again to let his words sink in. "Ya dangle upside down in your straps and get a canopy full of earth."

He simulated dangling from the five-point harness, in an inverted plane, with his eyes large and his hands grasping an imaginary stick in total terror.

His eyes locked with mine, "Then it pulls out."

The Navy test pilot smiled somewhat maliciously.

"Best ride I ever had."

A week or so after Engen and Ivans died, I was flying a Nimbus 4DM over Minden.

"I can show you what happened," my co-pilot friend offered, as if I needed an aerial lesson on unrecoverable situations, particularly after this accident.

He started a turn, to demonstrate the fatal error.

My throat closed; my breath quickened. I felt trapped inside the cockpit as a deep unease enveloped me. Panic started to eat away at my presence. Panicking in an airplane is not a smart idea.

"Let's not do this," I declared, my voice unsteady.

My friend must have sensed my extreme discomfort. "Your stick," he called.

And in that second, as pilot in command, my panic vanished. The cockpit seemed normal again. I was in control.

Which brings me to the question of what is control?

Control is something I've grappled with. It can give us a sense of self determination. It can drive us. It can even control us. It's both an illusion and seemingly real. I think the reason this incident so disturbed me is that it highlighted that exquisite balance between risk and reward, and the illusion of control that goes with it. I had to ask myself where I stood in that continuum.

I have definitely danced on the dark side of the sky. I've flown (unintentionally) into a rapidly developing thunderstorm that nearly killed me as I encountered violent up and down drafts that exceeded the Vne of my plane, with lightning strikes searing through the sky off my right wing. I've skimmed the tops of mountain ranges, trading altitude for daring speed.

I've also mourned too many aviation deaths. I once counted twenty-five deaths during a relatively short period. Some I knew personally, some I didn't. But each death touched me. The soaring community is small, and there are perhaps one or two degrees of separation between most of us. And we are all bound by our love for the sport.

Our love of the sport comes from the privilege of riding the energy of the Earth to soar long distances. Soaring is a humbling and spiritual experience. It's an intense, alternate reality that imparts confidence, skill, and joy. It offers wisdom if we are wise enough to listen.

Perhaps the lesson of this terrible crash that killed two luminaries in the soaring world isn't about control at all. Perhaps it's about recognizing risk and still choosing to live fully. Perhaps it's about the choice of living in love or living in fear. I love to fly. Sometimes I'm fearful. I wrestle with the contradiction, particularly after events like this. My answer is to get back in the cockpit and fly.

Control, I have decided, is an illusion. A powerful illusion, but one that ultimately gives way as life goes on. Perhaps the only reality is to be truly, intensely present; to have the courage to follow your heart, to find your bliss, to live in joy, and to attempt to soar, wherever that may take you.

And that brings me to the story of Chris Dahl-Bredine.

Meet My Guest, Chris Dahl-Bredine: Artist, Pilot, Photographer

Chris Dahl-Bredine's photographs can leave you breathless. Flying his trike, a home built ultralight that he calls a flying motorcycle, he captures the beauty and perspective of the Earth from the sky.

Chris dreamed of flying for years, but it was an incident in 1999 that sent him in that direction. Caught in an avalanche at Taos Ski Area, he tumbled down and over the mountain, breaking his back and arm. Suddenly his mortality seemed very real.

As I slowly recovered, I re-evaluated my life. The biggest thing I came away with was that I wanted to live more fully and follow my wildest dreams.

With a sudden recognition that our time here is so short, Chris started researching his dream of flying.

In his garage he built his trike; an experimental, open-air aircraft that would become his passport to flight. He developed his photography skills. And he explored.

His expeditions led him from the stunning mountains of Taos and Northern New Mexico into Colorado and Utah. Wildlife, rivers, and tributaries viewed from above gave him a new look at the interconnectedness of this world we inhabit.

Flying changed his life. It gave him a reason to mend beyond a broken back and sent him on a search for deeper meaning in his life. This is Chris's story.

Chris Dahl-Bredine: The Conversation

This conversation has been edited, but there's so much more to the story! When you have time, scan the QR code and you can listen to the original unedited conversation and view videos and photos of each guest. Or just visit BumpInTheRoad.us/Readers-Portal/ and sign in.

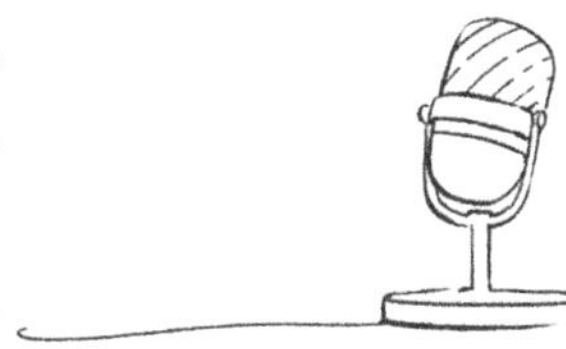

Chris: I moved to Towson, New Mexico when I just turned twenty and had an obsession and love for skiing. I was always so enthralled by anything that gave you the sense of flying, whether it was skiing or surfing; anything where you felt free from the bounds of gravity.

I had thought about flying since I was a kid. I wanted to be a pilot. When I was thirteen, I went up for a flight in Silver City with a local pilot. It was a really rough day.

It was an amazing experience, but I actually got motion sickness. I felt really discouraged because I thought maybe I wasn't cut out for this.

So, I put that dream on the back burner for a long time.

But I kept seeing hang gliders and these other ways of flying. I wanted to experience that freedom.

As long as I can remember, I had really vivid dreams about flying. And when I woke up, I just felt so alive.

For many years, skiing in fresh powder was a great substitute for flying. It's the closest thing to flying that I knew. But when I was around thirty, I was skiing up in Taos Ski Valley. There was two feet of fresh snow, and I was skiing in an area that hadn't been skied much. Before I knew it, I felt the whole mountain start to move with me.

I realized immediately I was in an avalanche,
and it was taking me right toward a cliff.

I tried everything I could to stop. I tried to grab a tree. I tried to just brace my skis into the snow. But it just took me, like I was a little feather floating on the surface of the snow, and pushed me right off of this forty-foot cliff head first.

I hit my skis on the rocks at the top of the cliff. I remember thinking, that's it, I'm done. I'm dead. And then I don't remember what happened for a while. My first memory after that was sitting in the snow up to my neck.

One of my friends was talking to me. I slowly started to remember what had happened. I just couldn't believe I was alive. I knew I had broken some bones. It felt like my wrist was broken and my back was definitely injured. I just sat there, kind of stunned and dazed and amazed that I was still alive.

It turned out that I had fractured my T9 vertebra. It wasn't a bad fracture, thankfully, because they didn't have to do surgery, but I was in pain for a long time. I started to realize that we could be gone any day, and every day was such a blessing to be alive.

Was I living the way I really dreamed of and really wanted to?

I realized I hadn't been listening to some of my dreams. And one of those dreams was flying. So, as I recovered, I started researching hang gliders and flying with this new enthusiasm and gratitude for being alive.

My research led me to a "trike." It's basically a hang glider wing on a three-wheel carriage with a motor. You can actually take off and land like an airplane. As soon as I saw those, I thought that would be really cool, because you don't have to jump off a mountain like you do with a hang glider; you can actually fly places and travel and you get to see everything from a total unobstructed view. After a year or so in recovery, I found a flight school in Arizona and booked a week of training with them.

I learned in the two-seater, but I had a similar experience as when I had flown when I was thirteen. It was very rough air and I started getting sick. I almost walked away and said, "I can't do this."

And then I went out on an evening flight when it was smooth as glass. There was a beautiful sunset. The whole sky lit up. And that's when I realized that I don't have to fly when the air is rough. There are certain times of the day and certain days when it's smooth. So,

I bought a used trike, came home with it, and started flying as often as I could back here in New Mexico.

Pat: Flying is certainly magical. Did you know that you wanted something that would be open to the air from the get go? Or did you consider a small plane or anything different?

Chris: Well, I had flown in a small plane and I just felt kind of separated from everything. I was looking out a little window and I really knew after I did that flight when I was thirteen, that

I wanted to fly something open so I could just be immersed in the sky . . .and see everything below me and all around me and feel the air. And so that's why I decided that this trike, this powered hang glider, would be the best thing.

Pat: It gives you amazing autonomy being able to take off and land on your own and not be dependent on anybody else. And you have a pretty good range. What, about five or six hundred miles?

Chris: Well, not quite, it depends on which wing you have on there. I have different speed wings, but I think with my faster wing, I probably have a 400-mile range more or less, depending on the wind.

Pat: Do you usually try to fly in the morning or evening when the air's a little bit calmer?

Chris: Yes. I still, to this day, even after almost twenty years of flying, don't like rough air.

Pat: I come at it from the opposite perspective, flying sailplanes. I love rough air. That's my energy.

Chris: I know. I've actually gotten much more tolerant to it than I used to be, but if it's rough for a long period, I start feeling queasy again. So, a lot of the year I end up flying early mornings between half an hour before sunrise and two or three hours after sunrise.

Pat: When did the photography come into the picture?

Chris: Even after the first couple of flights, you're so blown away by what you see, especially after being on land your whole life, you just want to share it with people. I had dabbled in photography, and I had a few cameras. As soon as I started feeling comfortable, I started bringing a camera with me and

every morning there was something new and beautiful to witness.

Pat: Your photography is beyond stunning. It's so beautiful. (Please check out some of Chris's photography on the website and on his Instagram account @ShotsFromAbove). What sort of avenues has this opened for you?

Chris: It's been an interesting road. I really want to convey the feeling of the freedom you have and the landscapes you're seeing.

First, it was film, because back then digital wasn't really that great. I went to medium format film, but I was limited by the number of pictures you could take in a flight because I had to change film manually. So, when digital got really good, I switched over. It was so much easier to be able to take a thousand pictures on a flight instead of thirty-five.

Pat: What are the advantages of shooting from a platform like your trike versus drone photography?

Chris: Well,

I think the main advantage is just the joy you get out of actually being up there.

While you're actually immersed in the subject that you're shooting, you can get angles that you wouldn't necessarily see through a screen of a drone. And you can go much further. You can cover two or three hundred miles of beautiful terrain shooting pictures, whereas a drone is limited to half an hour or so.

Pat: What was one of the more frightening aerial situations you ever ran into?

Chris: Well, as you know, the more you fly, the more chances you have of having some scary experiences. I would say probably the scariest one was having my engine die when I was flying over a mountain canyon and having to land very unexpectedly and very quickly on a highway with traffic on it.

That was really scary. And I gotta say when that happened, that was kind of like the avalanche experience in a way, because I was so shaken by it.

I really questioned everything I was doing and wondered, like why am I doing this? What is motivating me to do this? And do I really want to take this risk?

I just stewed on it for a long time. And what I came up with is that I really love what I'm doing and if I can use that experience to be safer, then that's what I would do.

So that was another bump in the road, the kind that takes you to the brink and makes you question everything in your life.

And then you can decide again, is this really what you want to do? And I decided, yes, it was. I love just being up there and I love sharing this perspective with the world.

I photograph the landscapes in New Mexico, Colorado, and Utah. Utah is such an alien landscape that it's hard to even fathom what you're seeing. I love just packing up and going for a multi-day or weeklong flying trip with everything I need in the trike and camping out. And to me that's one of the most invigorating, exciting things that I know of.

Pat: What sort of advice would you give to somebody on following your passion?

Chris: I think it's important to follow your passion, but I think at the same time, you have to realize that you are putting yourself into a whole different world that involves risks and that they have to be taken seriously, with lots of study and thought and practice and caution.

I would advise anyone to approach it slowly, really use your intuition, and don't rush into anything. Don't feel like you have to be in a hurry. Just let it unfold naturally to where you feel comfortable and you feel empowered as you do this, instead of feeling like you're pushing it.

I feel like you can fly safely if you do it right. If you feel comfortable and you feel energized by it, then you're doing it right. If you feel scared all the time and you kind of cringe when you think about it, then you're doing something wrong. I think it's really just staying in tune with yourself, with the weather, and with your aircraft.

Pat: I think flying really connects you to the Earth and to the world in a way that few things do. I mean the energy of the sky, the beauty. It's just such an incredible experience. What life lessons would you pass along from your time in the air?

Chris: There are so many positive things I've taken from these experiences. I think when you see how everything is so interconnected on the planet and you see how we are so interconnected to all the systems of the planet just to stay alive. . .

You realize we're all in this together.

And I think those kinds of connections are important as we move forward, because we need to connect on a more global scale if we want to keep healthy life on Earth going. I feel like we're at a point where we've lived in a disconnected way with our society and with each other and that it's not serving us. And the more we can build those connections again, we can learn how to thrive in harmony with each other and with the Earth in a way that's sustainable.

Thoughts for You to Ponder

What dream have you put on the backburner?

How does that dream make you feel? Happy, elated, energized?

What's more powerful: the emotion of your dream or the energy that's holding you back?

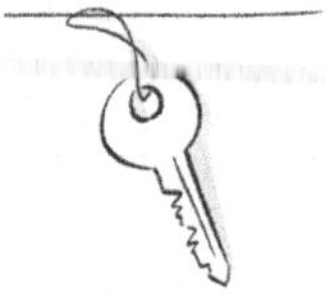

Key Takeaways

- Even if control is an illusion, you do control your thoughts and your responses
- Your thoughts and responses create your reality
- Your reality can be your dream

CHAPTER SIX

A City Boy Meets the Appalachian Trail

"Nature started teaching me about myself."

–JESSE CODY

It is in the silence of nature we so often learn to see things more clearly. Our mind stills, we connect to our bodies, and we reconnect with the natural rhythm of the Earth. Nature is experiential and touches us in a place beyond our minds and in our souls.

Some of our best metaphors come from the outdoors: to climb a mountain, to cast a line, to walk a path. They speak to the timeless human need to make a tangible connection with the intangible. There is something about the very presence, the essence of nature, that speaks silently to that need.

Nature is one of my companions. She challenges me, makes me think, and sometimes she just takes my breath away. Her wisdom introduces me to experiences beyond this place and time. She is greater than anything I can imagine, yet I am one with her.

In this chapter, nature offers a glimpse into a deeper realm of understanding and existence, both for me and for my guest, Jesse Cody.

Lake Tahoe, 1999

Incline Village, Nevada, sits on the northern shore of Lake Tahoe providing a view that stretches as far as the eye can see. It's an amazing place to kayak, to hike, and to soar. The combination resonates deeply with my soul.

In the outdoors, I find peace and a transcendent truth that I'm not sure I fully understand. There is something about the impossible scale and majesty that is humbling and inspiring all at once. It opens an indefinable avenue of timeless peace and connection, as I found flying over Lake Tahoe one summer afternoon:

Sun streamed through the canopy. It was brilliant, warm, and enveloping. The sky was blue and below the sapphire-turquoise waters of Tahoe laid like a jewel on the Earth.

I sat in the cockpit, a thin fiberglass shell held aloft by fifteen meters of flexing wing. At the edge of each wing was a small winglet that projected vertically into the sky.

I banked the plane, the tiny winglet parallel with the Earth, searching for lift.

I felt lift under the winglet. It was a bubble of air and I balanced on it. The plane and I were one. Together we rose—we danced—into the sky.

Warm sun streamed through the cockpit.
Endless blue sky; Tahoe below.

It was a moment of perfect synchronicity.
The energy of the air, the warmth of the sun,
the beauty of the earth.

And for that timeless moment, all was one.

Sun, energy, beauty. And I was riding in the midst
of it all, connected to it all, then and forever.

This moment has stayed with me, and its intensity hasn't diminished with time. It's an experience that gave me a sense of knowing that is rooted in the unknowable. It's a window into eternity. And that experience, that knowing, lives within me.

There is a purity in nature that is deeply inspiring. But it is not without its harsh edges. In the air, violent updrafts and downdrafts can threaten the structural integrity of your plane until the storm passes. On the ground, fire and earthquakes can quickly ravage all that man has built. But afterwards comes the healing, the land reassembles, the forest regrows, man rebuilds, and the Earth goes on.

Somewhere, I was looking for that secret of continuity and growth. I still stung from the rejection of divorce. I was still unsettled, having lost all my connections to my prior life. I realized I needed to heal and move on, but I didn't know how. So, I looked to nature hoping I would find whatever it was I was looking for. So did Jesse Cody.

Meet My Guest, Jesse Cody: Mental Health Warrior, Outdoorsman

Jesse Cody has made the outdoors his passion and his raison d'etre. His drive towards nature grew out of a period of deep dissatisfaction and depression. He was desperate for a life of meaning.

But to find it, he needed a change. So it was that this city boy (New York and Boston) headed off into the wilderness to hike the Appalachian Trail. Jesse had never pitched a tent, walked any significant distance, or spent time alone in the outdoors.

Tackling the Appalachian Trail as a hiking novice, Jesse realized that the trail would be a challenge. Only 25 percent finished the 2,200-mile hike, and Jesse's hiking experience was nil. But in the woods, step by step, he found peace.

Hiking uplifted my spirit and convinced me that life was worth living.

I was finally able to calm the voices in my head that I'd spent a lifetime battling and actually engage with them from a thoughtful and grounded place.

"Hike the good hike" became his mantra.

Jesse credits his quest with saving his life, and now he is saving the lives of others.

Jesse Cody: The Conversation

This conversation has been edited, but there's so much more to the story! When you have time, scan the QR code and you can listen to the original unedited conversation and view videos and photos of each guest. Or just visit BumpInTheRoad.us/Readers-Portal/ and sign in.

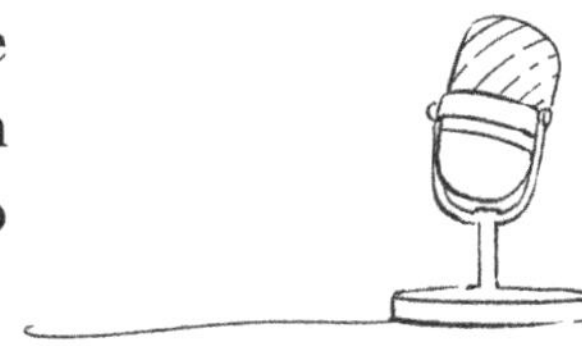

Jesse: My name is Jesse Cody. I'm the founder of Hike the Good Hike. I focus on using hiking and wilderness exploration to improve mental health.

For many years, I struggled with my own mental health. And I tried to do it on my own without seeking out help.

I was in my mid- to late-thirties. I battled depression and major insecurity issues. I just felt completely lost in life, and all that came together in thoughts of suicide. I felt that I didn't want to be here anymore. Then I turned forty.

My friends and family put together a big party for me. I can remember thinking that this might be my last birthday. And then, in the moment of the birthday party, there was this recognition of love surrounding me. There were so many people there to celebrate me.

"How can one think about ending their life when they have so much good in their life?" I thought about that for a couple of days.

I realized that I hadn't explored all the avenues that one should explore when they're battling such incredible demons. I made the decision that I wanted to live, but I didn't know how. And if I was going to live, I had to figure out how to live with purpose.

I wanted to embrace life, but I didn't know how to do that.

I was strictly a city guy. At the age of forty, I'd spent the majority of my life in Boston and New York City, working in the restaurant industry. I was also battling narcissistic behavior and taking advantage of my staff. I was drinking heavily.

I started recognizing that there were a lot of things that I had to change about myself. I was going to have to figure out a new path.

I had to take a break, recharge, and figure out how I could restart my life.

What did I do? Should I go back to school? Should I fall back on things that I had done in my early twenties, before restaurant management? I had no clue what to do.

Trying to restart your life at forty is just as scary as suicidal thoughts.

But then I came across an article written about Robert Redford, who was making Bill Bryson's book, *A Walk in the Woods*, into a movie. I had read this book in my early twenties. It's about hiking the Appalachian Trail. It was about someone who was trying to figure out what his purpose was in life.

It was at chapter two that a light bulb flicked on.

I said to myself, I think I could use a long walk.

Now, obviously, as someone who knew nothing about the wilderness, thinking about 2,200 miles from Georgia to Maine was a bit daunting. It was a leap, a big crazy leap, but what did I have to lose? I was suicidal. I was ready to do whatever it took.

So, the decision to hike the Appalachian Trail was made.

People accepted it, but they laughed. They claimed I'd be back in a week.

I put my life in a backpack and jumped on a train on March 14, 2015, down to Georgia. On March 15, I found myself on Springer Mountain. And I started walking.

The walk that saved my life.

It took me six months. I walked every step of it. And on September 15, six months to the day, I summited Mount Katahdin and became a true hiker of the Appalachian Trail. I don't think I can ever say that out loud and not get emotional, knowing that I accomplished something like that.

Pat: What did you encounter on the trail?

Jesse: I encountered a lot of things. I didn't go into the hike fit. I was out of shape. I knew that the first month to month and a half was going to be physically difficult.

My whole life was living in a tent out of a backpack. The first time I had ever set up and slept in a tent was night one of the Appalachian Trail. I was really a rookie.

Pat: I know from experience that setting up a tent is not always easy.

Jesse: It's not. And then there's cooking on the littlest stove you've ever seen. There goes the free cheeseburgers and fries that I had at the restaurants I was managing.

It was going to be peanut butter and ramen noodles for a long time.

My mind kept saying, "Why do you think you can do this? You can't do this. You're not cut out for this."

But I just went in with this complete understanding that everything was going to be a challenge.

At that point in 2015, more than 70 percent of the people that attempted the Appalachian Trail dropped out.

I knew the odds were against me, but up until that point, the odds for life were against me, too. I knew from day one that I wasn't going to quit. I was tired of quitting.

Pat: From a mental health perspective, what sort of evolution did you see? Because there's a lot of time to think and reflect and to deal with the voices that we all have in our heads.

Jesse: Going in, I knew the hike was going to try to break me. That's what it's there for.

I also started understanding that once I made the decision to live, that I needed guidance. This is the point where the universe and Mother Nature came together and said, "Now that he's found the ability to want to stay with us, let's take him by the hand and guide him."

I could almost hear the wilderness saying to me, "Don't think this is going to be easy. We're going to make you earn every single step of this. But if you do it, you're going to find your way out of your darkness."

It also made me understand that you don't get cured of mental health illness. What you do is challenge yourself and come to an understanding with the voices.

For so long, I lived in chaos. Everywhere was chaos. Bars, cities, my surroundings.

But on the trail, even the voices in my mind were overcome with these new surroundings of mine, this beauty, this quietness. Nature is just such an amazing place to have conversations when there's very little noise around you. But in the noise is such incredible beauty, whether it's birds, whether it's the wind, whether it's your feet, just crushing pine needles as you walk forward.

Since 2015, I've spent the majority of my life in the wilderness.

There's never a moment that I'm not in awe.

It hits me every day. And it gives me the strength and the ability to truly work with these voices in my head and let them know that I love life. And you're not going to take that away from me.

Pat: In the wilderness, did you miss the hustle and bustle or was it sort of an immediate sense of this is where I belong? Did you go through a bit of withdrawal?

Jesse: It was an immediate sense of this is where I belong. It started teaching me about myself. It opened me. It made me more open-minded and much less judgmental of people and things and the way that life should be.

When I was a restaurant bar manager, I was a stubborn little city guy who liked sports. And if you walked in my bar, and you dressed differently, I was probably judging you before you even opened your mouth.

But on the trail, you come across so many different types of people that you may never have spoken to before. You start having conversations and you start to get an understanding of what their life is about.

You get an understanding of why they're on trail.

You start seeing things that are similar and you start appreciating the things that are different.

The trail started chipping away at my narcissism and criticism. I was in a state of awe, and through that came empathy and a lot of love. I felt love constantly.

The trail was bringing out the best in me. It was creating things and showing me things that I could be. With the excitement, the emotion, I finally started figuring out that I was right for this place, that I was right for life.

Pat: What happened after you finished the Appalachian Trail?

Jesse: I knew coming off the trail, that's when withdrawal was going to kick in. What did I do now? I had to go back to the Boston area. I had to get a job. What kind of job was I going to get?

I came off the trail knowing that I was going to build towards the life that I wanted.

I had started saying a mantra very early on while hiking the Appalachian Trail, which is

Hike the good hike.

I was just so incredibly happy that I wanted to live. I thought, "This is too good to keep to yourself. This has to be shared. You must find a way to share your story."

I knew that there were probably a ton of people out there that shared my story. We witness suicide on a daily basis. So many people just don't know where to turn.

I had been blogging while on the trail. I knew that I could use social media and build this movement. Everything that I was going to do when I got off the Appalachian Trail was going to be focused toward building Hike the Good Hike.

I'm approaching ten thousand miles hiking since my first steps off Springer Mountain on the Appalachian Trail, and I'm becoming a nonprofit.

I want to use my hiking to raise money and awareness for other programs. This July 1, I am partnering with a nonprofit organization out of New England called the Youth Mental Health Project. I'm going to be using the last 1,300 miles of the Pacific Crest Trail starting on July 1 to bring awareness to mental health and to fundraise for their organization.

Pat: Wow. That's great. Mental health is something that is such a serious issue. I was doing a little digging around on the web the other day, and I was stunned by some of the statistics. One out of five Americans in any given year is dealing with mental illness. That's astonishing.

Jesse: If that's not a cry for help, I don't know what is.

Pat: There's a stigma associated with a lot of mental health issues and that's unfair.

Jesse: The stigma is alarming. So many young adults, young men, are afraid that they're going to be judged for being depressed.

It took me over forty years to speak up. I didn't tell my family and friends that I was suicidal until two years after I finished the Appalachian Trail. I was still in that place where I was embarrassed to say it out loud.

Pat: And what kind of reaction did you get from them?

Jesse: You just think there's going to be so much negativity coming from saying that out loud, whereas, in reality, you're probably going to get a positive reaction.

It's a weight off your shoulders. When I was able to finally say I was suicidal, I remember this massive breath came out of me.

I could finally be honest about where I was.

Pat: I'm going to take a slight tangent here. I want to read something that you wrote that I just loved, and I think it occurred when you were hiking White Sands. You wrote,

Beauty is what the land breathes into me, life.
It's a constant reminder to me, a man who not so
long ago did not believe life was worth living.

Jesse: I've come a long way. Because six, seven years ago there was just this constant thought all the time about wanting to end my life. And so, whether it's White Sands, Great Sands, Yosemite, or whatever trail I'm hiking, I always take the moment to just kind of let my surroundings embrace me.

Pat: Nature is so powerful. It's beautiful. It's overwhelming, it's threatening. And I think most of all, it puts us in our place in a good way.

Jesse: I was just up in New Mexico the other day I got this crazy photograph of a lightning bolt. You couldn't see the lightning bolt, but you could see the flashes and the clouds over the mountains. And I thought to myself how little we are to this big, big world. And then if you can't just kick back and take it all in and realize that you're missing out.

Open your eyes, really open your eyes.

Pat: You've given up a traditional life, which isn't easy to do in our society. What advice would you have for somebody considering something along those lines?

Jesse: You must understand that you've got to really simplify your life. Sell off a lot of your stuff. Put some stuff in storage. For me, for the most part, if I'm not hiking, I am traveling in my vehicle, which I sleep out of. It gives me the ability to get to a lot of amazing, beautiful places. I pick up odd jobs here and there, mostly bartending.

It's about paying attention to what it does for your mind and your soul than what society tells us should be your life.

There are moments when I'm lonely. This can be a very lonely way of living, even though I have all this beauty around me. I have to keep my eye on the big picture of what I'm trying to accomplish. And I have to believe that it will lead to good things.

If I keep working hard with Hike the Good Hike
it will provide whatever it's supposed to provide.

I have a belief system that believes in nature and the universe. They came and got me when I decided I wanted to live. And they have a plan for me.

Thoughts For You to Ponder

Do you ever feel like there is a disconnect between your public and private self? How would you characterize it?

What would it take for your public and private selves to sync up?

Where in your life do you feel most connected, that you are "hiking the good hike?"

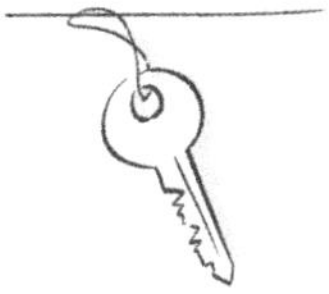

Key Takeaways

- Your mental health is so important; it needs to be a priority
- Nature has the power to heal, transform, and bring peace to our lives
- Simplicity offers riches that things cannot

CHAPTER SEVEN

Daring to Create the Life You Long For

"What people don't realize is that sometimes you're risking more by not by not listening to yourself."

–TAMA KIEVES

What happens when you live a life not true to yourself? You may present the confidence that goes with a "perfect life," but what happens when something inside you screams for a different path? How do you define it, much less understand it? And how do you realize it?

Finding congruence between a soulful path and so-called reality can be challenging. It's usually a disconnect between your inner knowing and your outer world. And the only way to reconcile the two is to go within; to seek your truth. Only by going within can you find that path forward. And chances are it will be a bumpy ride.

Reno/Tahoe, Nevada, 2015

My kitchen flooded while I was out of town. Restoring the house meant emptying the kitchen's contents and moving to a nearby townhouse while the work was done.

As I emptied the cabinets, box after box was filled. Dual bowl ice cream makers, multiple Cuisinarts, French and Italian plates, long stemmed glasses, and beautiful Italian silverware sets. A juicer, a blender or two, and endless serving paraphernalia. The boxes were stacked, floor to ceiling, in the guest room.

Where had all this stuff come from?

I was appalled at the sheer volume of *things*. I assured myself that they were devices of culinary creativity, not just a random pile of pots and pans. But I had hit a tipping point. What was the point of all of this?

Meanwhile in the townhouse, I lived minimally. Months passed, the insurance company dragged their feet, but eventually the restoration was complete.

I remember driving up the hill into the development where I lived. The Sierra was still frosted in winter snow, and in the valley, the crabapple and pear trees were starting to bloom. It was spring, traditionally a time of renewal. But something was amiss. I could feel it. What should have been a welcoming drive home felt strangely foreboding.

I tried to slough off this malaise, but something had changed. Or perhaps I had. But whatever the disconnect, it eluded me, and I went back to life as usual, puttering to put my perfect house back in perfect order. My life was happy. Or was it?

In my heart I knew that something wasn't right. Little did I know that this malaise was the harbinger of yet another major life change that would send me on a quest for what *was* right.

And so it was for my guest, Kama Kieves, whose quest for her soul sent her in a most unexpected direction.

Meet My Guest, Tama Kieves: Harvard Lawyer, Coach

How might a Harvard Law degree change your life? Would you be wealthy? Famous? Well regarded?

Tama Kieves graduated with honors from Harvard Law and landed a prestigious job. But it didn't make her happy, and ultimately, she walked away from it all with no clear idea of what might lie ahead.

So, she began a new life; a life of reacquainting herself with who she really was. It was a non-linear path toward her real dream, which was to write.

I just couldn't find my way in the world.
I had to find myself first.

Tama spent the first eleven years after leaving her corporate job essentially finding herself.

If I had to tell you just one thing about thriving through uncertainty, I'd tell you this:

Do whatever it takes to discover, connect, and
deepen your relationship to your Inspired Self.

Life, Tama realized, wasn't linear.

Linear institutions celebrate left-brain achievement; our society celebrates external and material achievement. Is it any wonder it's so hard to find and follow our hearts?

Living an inspired life is more of an evolution than a revolution. It unfolds over time, with each small step building on the previous one. Tama's not suggesting that you leave your job. Rather, you look within to see what inspires you and start to integrate it into your current life. It's a life-long process that is both challenging and rewarding.

The level of consciousness that creates the problem is not the level of consciousness that can give birth to a solution.

We're talking about a creative, inspired journey.

Tama Kieves: The Conversation

This conversation has been edited, but there's so much more to the story! When you have time, scan the QR code and you can listen to the original unedited conversation and view videos and photos of each guest. Or just visit BumpInTheRoad.us/Readers-Portal/ and sign in.

Pat: Tama, you have an incredible story about having a Harvard law degree, a job to die for, and you walked away from it all. Can you tell us a little bit about that?

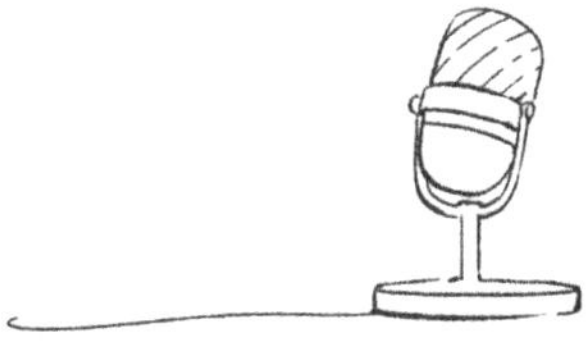

Tama: It was the most important decision of my lifetime. I think I represent a lot of people in that I knew a little bit of who I was when I was young, but I didn't listen to it. When I was growing up, I knew that I loved to write. I grew up in a Brooklyn, New York, Orthodox Jewish household, and so if you said you wanted to write, it was:

If you are going to write, you're going to starve.

So that was it and I went off to law school. I got accepted to Harvard Law School and graduated with honors. Many of us think that you have to stay reasonable, you have to stay practical, you have to deny what you love.

I ended up practicing law in a major law firm, doing well, and just feeling emptier and emptier and emptier in a scary way. What was I doing with my life?

I was terrified because I had what you're supposed to have in terms of American success.

But I just felt devastated inside because I wasn't doing something that meant anything to me. I remember being so unhappy, and a friend of mine at the time said:

Think about it, if you've been this successful doing something you don't love, what could you do with what you love?

And that made sense to me on a logical level. I was so unhappy, and I just thought:

You get one lifetime.

That's what began my entire journey. I walked out of my law firm without a plan, without anything, and just thinking, "I've got to at least try this."

And that's become my life's work, to help other people listen to their inner instincts with whatever transitions or changes they're going through.

Pat: Do you think you were driven more by getting away from your unhappiness, or towards another happiness?

Tama: Oh, what a great question. A little bit of both. I think sometimes the unhappiness that we have is so great because there is this inner brightness, or inner light, or inner instinct of something we deeply want that we're burying and squelching and denying.

I think at the time it was just survival. I had to get out of there or I was going to die. But I think there was also that whisper of there's got to be something more.

Pat: The uncertainty you face with that kind of decision can be paralyzing. How did you push through that?

Tama: Still pushing through it. Actually, pushing is probably not the right word. Pushing is what my inner control freak instincts would do, but

This has been a path of unlearning a linear, pushing, aggressive force way of thinking and learning how to listen to love; learning how to listen to an inner instinct or a whisper and not to push.

I think for me, the thing that was most life-changing was adopting a spiritual path, and I was the least likely person to go that way. For me, it was a *Course in Miracles*, which is a path of living in love instead of fear.

I have come to see uncertainty as opportunity.

It's an opportunity for pain, misery, and exhaustion or it's an opportunity for extraordinary choices. My latest book is *Thriving Through Uncertainty*, and the premise of that book is that uncertainty is going to be here, and when uncertainty happens, it's our opening; it's our moment to finally listen to something else that's inside us because all the old ways aren't working. All the things we know, all the things we've tried, they're not working in the traditional ways.

And so, finally, we might be available to open to this extraordinary voice that's inside us.

It's not a linear path, it's an inspired path.

Pat: You have some Albert Einstein quotes in your book, which I love. I'm a fan of his quotes. And one of the ones I really like is, "It is better to believe than to disbelieve. In doing so, you bring everything into the realm of possibility."

Tama: Absolutely. When I think about my own life, I knew I wanted to write. But I did not believe in that possibility. I was told that possibility was crazy, I would starve, I could never make it. My own healing has been in learning how to believe in possibilities.

Many of us have gone through a few bumps, and it's very easy and understandable to close our hearts down, to stop believing. As a writer, I've had eight billion rejections. I've had so many things that didn't work. Same thing with being a speaker. I have many rational reasons to have stopped.

I am not interested in rational reasons.
I am interested in inspiration and genius and love.

It is in my choosing to dare again and believe again that opened my heart, my love, my sanity, and my deepest capacities. It's given me the life I dreamed of. I believe we're here in this lifetime to constantly keep our hearts open, our minds open, and be willing to dare again.

Pat: I think it's the only approach to take, to be true to yourself, to your soul, and really find your path in life. But it's a huge jump for so many people because it goes against the societal grain. Society values that left brain external and material achievement. What car do you drive? Where do you live? It's no wonder that it's so hard for people to find and follow their hearts. How do you separate yourself from that very thin materialistic veneer that many of us think is real?

Tama: It's tough.

It's this consistent choice of what I call linear success versus inspired success.

Linear success is exactly what you just described, where there's prescribed standards, you go to the right school, you get the right degree, you get the right job, the right car, the right look.

For me, inspired success is being moved from within; being moved moment by moment. And for many of us, we've done the linear success model.

I did all the "right things" and I felt empty. It was terrifying.

My own healing has been learning that there's the appearance of what life looks like, but then there's the experience, and the experience of being alive. I'm much more interested in creating a meaningful life.

We're so caught up in a material society; you have to have this now, you have to have that now.

We're so busy going and going and going that we can't even feel our hearts.

We can't feel what we want. We don't even know what we want.

I want to find out what your dream is, not what you're supposed to dream.

It takes so much courage to be an independent maverick soul that's daring to live the one life you are meant to live. I use a technique called the inspired self-dialogues, which is a journaling technique. I just write from my state of mind. It's just tapping into a different form of sanity when I need it.

Pat: It's actually tapping into your wiser self and you need your wiser self, because if you live that linear life, you supposedly know what the next step is, right? But if you live an inspired life, you're really living much more in the present moment and creating it step-by-step.

Tama: I always talk about it as following the breadcrumbs. I have a very linear, ambitious, crazy mind. So, this wasn't easy for me. What happens on this path is that a lot of my breadcrumbs led me to change the way I think, because:

The issue is never in what steps we take or how we get there.
The issue is always in the way we're thinking.

We limit ourselves with the way we're thinking, where we carry forward are these wounds and these issues and these negative attitudes that we all have.

Breadcrumbs are transformative. Your linear mind might fight it. I'll give a crazy example. When I was much younger, I met a man and I fell in love with him. He told me I might not want to date him because he was moving at the end of the summer.

In a linear mind, I was thinking he was right, don't get hurt. He was not the kind of guy my parents would approve of anyway. But I followed that energy, and I followed that instinct, and it was one of the most transformative relationships of my life.

He was a very free thinker and very creative and I hadn't been exposed to that at that time in my life. And it changed the way I thought. I remember him saying, "If you ever get a chance, go out west. It's amazing."

I filed that in my brain, and many, many years later, I moved to Denver, and it's been one of the best things I ever did.

That was a breadcrumb. It was not something from a linear path. It is a path of following energy, not rational thought.

Pat: Energy and your soul. One of the things that you say in your book is, "I just couldn't find my way in the world; I had to find myself first."

Tama: What I always tell people is that this is a path not so much of doing, but undoing and undoing again, those painful beliefs, those painful ways of not believing in yourself, and not trusting.

Not trusting that you have a soul, not trusting that there is a way, not trusting that there really is a love and a light and a force of good. Whatever you call it, the universe, God, spirit, or higher mind, whatever it is, follow something other than your fears, other than what you think is practical.

It was like learning a completely new language to find myself. I would never have dreamed that I would have anything to do with spirituality. It was not on my ticket, you know. I was in Harvard Law School.

Pat: What was the evolution of faith in your life?

Tama: That's an interesting question. Well, first, pure desperate freaking need is always a good motivation.

When I first left law, I was off the grid. Before, I'd found faith in my business card, in my sexy title, in my sexy suit, in my bank account. That was my faith. When all of that is stripped from you, you have to find faith in something else. I didn't necessarily believe in religion. I had come from the Jewish religion, but it just didn't make me feel connected.

But what did make me feel connected was when I started following something I loved. For me, it was writing. It felt like I tapped into something bigger.

I think that's what this journey is. It's about being more open and discovering who we really are by following what we really want. That's where we discover who we are. And most of us have so many capacities. We don't tap into them because we're trying so hard to fit into an image or an identity or story that we think is us.

Pat: One of the things you mentioned, too, is that your spirit craves growth. But growth comes with risk. It is so hard for most people to live in uncertainty or take risks. What percentage of people do you think are willing to take these sorts of risks?

Tama: Following an inner voice is a very nuanced prescription, and each of us is completely different. So, risk could be very different. It might not be walking out of a career, it might be staying there and growing, or it may be speaking up. I never want people to think, "Oh God, I couldn't do what she did."

You're not supposed to do what I did.

Pat: You're supposed to do what you need to do.

Tama: Exactly.

What people don't realize is that sometimes you're risking more by not listening to yourself.

So, I wanted to share with you just a few lines from *Thriving Through Uncertainty,* and it's one of my favorite quotes in it. I thought I'd just quote my own book now, what the hell!

You may feel like things are challenging at this moment in your life, but let's get this straight right now. It's not because you're failing or broken, it's because your spirit demands soaring, not coping. It's your time. It's like the poet Rumi said, "Why would you prefer to crawl when you've been given wings?"

Pat: I think the key is being open to your inner voice, open to evolution. One of my favorite Einstein quotes is, I'm paraphrasing a bit, but, "You can't solve a problem with the same energy that created it."

I think that's so true, but to evolve to a different energy, a nonlinear energy, an energy of hope and possibility, takes time. It does not happen overnight for most of us.

Tama: I love that quote. It's like the level of consciousness that creates the problem is not the level of consciousness that can give birth to a solution. And we're talking about a creative inspired journey.

We have different solutions and different capacities. Our brain chemistry is literally different. I think that if we study more about following energy, following what is working, following what does light us up, following different creative solutions, we will tap capacities and creativity that can solve things in ways we cannot possibly imagine.

I always tell my clients that we're not here to make it in the world; we're here to remake the world.

We are here to remake the world with our creativity and our possibility, new solutions, and new ways, and I deeply believe that's what's happening.

Pat: If you could rewrite your personal story, would you?

Tama: Oh God, that's a hard question.

Pat: It's an impossible question so any answer goes.

Tama: Yes, you know, I've thought about that a lot. I went to Harvard Law School, on the campus of Harvard. I've thought, "What if I'd gone there and studied writing and made all those connections for something I loved?"

But then, there's something that's so perfect about my life, about having gone down this one track that didn't work. Now it's become my life's mission to help other people find their way. And so that credential, that grand mistake, I wouldn't change it.

Thoughts For You to Ponder

What parts of your life are a creative, inspired journey?

How have family or societal expectations influenced your life?

If you just get this one life, what do you want to do with it?

Key Takeaways

- Don't be afraid to follow your heart
- Be open to your own evolution
- Life is so much greater than just material success; it's full of boundless possibilities

CHAPTER EIGHT

No Barriers

"It was saying yes to opportunities."

–ERIK WEIHENMAYER

Life is full of self-imposed barriers. But what if, as Erik Weihenmayer would say, "What's within us is stronger than what's in our way?"

Part of navigating a bump in the road is to bring fresh energy into your life, one step at a time. Sometimes it's difficult. We stumble. But each step forward is full of possibilities.

What you choose to do really doesn't matter. In time, the activity will sort itself out. It's about resisting the heaviness of indecision, about refusing to be sidelined, and about introducing new energy into your day-to-day existence. Successfully navigating a bump means letting go of the past and opening the door to something new and meaningful to you.

It requires an open mind and courage to walk through that doorway. No one epitomizes this better than Erik Weihenmayer. He is a person who sees no barriers and achieves what seems to be impossible. He is one of the most inspiring people I've ever met.

Calistoga, California, 1989

I was on a trip to consider changing my life. It had become apparent that my marriage was yesterday's news, even if it would take several more years of death throes to bring it to its inevitable end.

I was hurt. I was lost. I was alone. I found myself in northern California, visiting wineries and contemplating different ways of life. I enjoyed the beautiful country and followed the winding road up to the northern end of the Napa Valley to Calistoga. Shops and restaurants lined the main street.

I wandered and decided to stay for the evening. A pink neon hotel sign flashed, beckoning me inside into a cozy room overlooking the hotel grounds.

In the morning, after a fitful sleep, I poured a cup of hot black coffee down in the hotel dining room and headed out to the pool. I pulled my sweater close. The morning dew settled heavily on the grass. The heat from my coffee cup rose in thin wisps of warmth, the pool lapped lazily at the tile along its rim, and the morning sun spread across the hills bringing a warm golden light to the valley.

Calistoga, in 1989, was a sleepy town famous for its mud baths. I had no particular reason for being there. It was just another waypoint in my wanderings.

The town is a bit quirky in that an airport runway intersects with the main road through town. A sign alongside the runway advertises glider rides.

"Rides won't start 'til eleven or so," I was told by the gentleman in the run-down office where gray wood splintered through faded white paint.

Eleven. I had planned to head back to San Francisco, then onto L.A. to meet up with some friends. Maybe I'd move to California? I really had no idea where or what I was going to do with a new, unwanted, soon-to-be-solo life.

"Okay," I responded to the man at the airport. "I'll come back at eleven."

At the appointed hour, I returned. The airport was starting to bustle as the planes were prepared for the day's flights. I was introduced to my pilot, a retired gentleman who directed me to an old Schweitzer 233. I'd never seen such a strange plane. It was clunky and made of fabric. Would this thing really fly?

I settled into the cockpit with the pilot in the seat behind me. Shortly thereafter, in a haze of swirling dust and noise, we followed the tow plane into the air.

We soared over vineyards and hills. The rows of perfectly aligned grape vines snaked their way up and over the gentle valley hills. It was a beautiful clear day, and from our eagle's eye perch we could see for miles.

Eventually, we returned to the airport and landed. The experience didn't really impress me all that much. I paid my bill and headed back to San Francisco in my rented white Mustang convertible. The wind blew through my hair and the sun warmed my face. I was still without direction in my life, other than just to survive this divorce. And there on that winding road through wine country, I wondered what to do. Should I move? What might I like to do? San Francisco had plenty of opportunity. Flying was not part of my paradigm.

I didn't know it yet, but my willingness to somehow put one foot in front of the other, at a time when I felt hurt, abandoned, and alone, would lead me to places and experiences I never imagined. I would learn that I was brave, I was capable, and I could do previously unthinkable things. If there is one bit of wisdom that came from this seemingly innocuous glider ride, it is to be willing to simply say yes.

Meet My Guest, Erik Weihenmayer: Mountaineer, Kayaker, Inspirational Leader

Erik is the founder of NoBarriers.org. Their motto: "What's within you is stronger than what's in your way."

When Erik was in ninth grade, he lost his ability to see due to a rare disease, retinoschisis. His loss of sight translated into some very difficult years. Anger, confusion, and finally some degree of acceptance accompanied him as he learned to navigate a sightless world.

I had to just leave the sighted world behind.

At the age of sixteen, a rock-climbing trip changed Erik's life. The tangible nature of the rock, the challenge, and the ability to navigate through texture and feel inspired Erik. He had found something he loved; something outdoors and something he could do. It gave him a sense of freedom and possibility; a sense that his adventure was just beginning.

That glimpse of possibility inspired Erik. He may have lost his sight, but not his vision, and his world kept expanding. He would go on to climb Everest and all Seven Summits and to kayak, solo, through the daunting Colorado River rapids.

Erik has changed the way the blind and disabled communities are seen. But most importantly, he is changing the way people view their own lives and possibilities. Upon summitting Everest, Erik was told:

Don't let this be the greatest thing you ever do.

What does one say to such advice? And even more importantly, what did Erik do?

The Conversation: Erik Weihenmayer

This conversation has been edited, but there's so much more to the story! When you have time, scan the QR code and you can listen to the original unedited conversation and view videos and photos of each guest. Or just visit BumpInTheRoad.us/Readers-Portal/ and sign in.

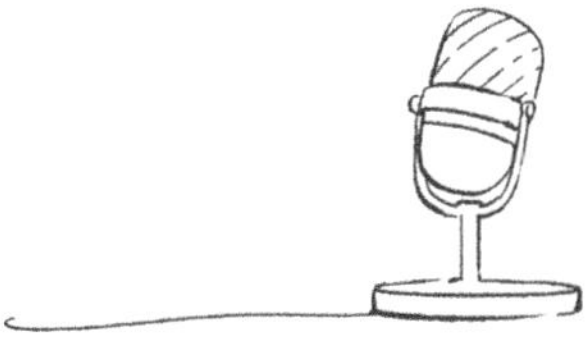

Erik: I was diagnosed with this very rare eye disease called retinoschisis probably at age four. One doctor out of Boston said I'd be blind by my early teens. And there was no cure.

I coped by just ignoring it, just going out and playing in the woods and trying to have fun with my friends. I wasn't allowed to do a lot of contact sports because if I got hit on the head, my retinas would detach even more.

I went blind about two weeks before my freshman year. My family was prepared for this. I was the only one unprepared. I thought, "Okay, this is real."

I didn't know how to describe it. It was like a baseball bat to the side of the head; that kind of just shock and finality of it all.

I was a frustrated, angry kid for a long time.

I grew up in Connecticut, and we'd have these raccoons that would come into our house. They'd break through our screened door. They'd eat our garbage and you'd sometimes come across them and you'd see their bright eyes. And they'd just be snarling at you from the corner. And I was basically that raccoon for a long time, just snarling at the world.

Pat: That breaks your heart to even think of it. But I think anger is a natural reaction for all of us when something like this happens.

Erik: Yeah. And it wasn't like the kind of angry, like yelling at people. It was more just withdrawing. I didn't want anybody to help me. I hated the way people perceived me.

For example, walking through the hallway, kids wouldn't know how to react to me. I felt like an egg that had cracked in the middle of the hall and there was yoke spilling everywhere and people were kind of just stepping around it. I'm not trying to make the audience feel sorry for me or anything, but I had a group of good friends that I'd play with when I could see. And I guess they were embarrassed for me, just because they didn't know how to react. And I didn't know how to react, either.

I was bitter and resentful. I remember one kid at this table with a group of kids. He just said, "shhh," and everyone would get really quiet so I wouldn't know they were there. I heard them breathing and I just said, "Screw you guys!"

I walked on and sat at a table by myself.

There were a lot of really big changes for me at that point, where I felt really isolated.

There was this bridge between me and the rest of the world, and I did not know how to get back into the world.

Pat: How did you get back?

Erik: It's not like there's this perfectly neat formula that you'd have on a motivational poster. Hope was not killed in my heart. I wanted to do things. So:

Whenever I had opportunities to do things, I would do them.

I got a letter in braille from a group taking blind kids on these recreational trips. One time they took us rock climbing.

It was such an adventure for me, scanning with my hands and feet, using them as my eyes, mapping out the rock and problem solving my way up the base. I was a very physical kid and I loved it. It was everything I thought adventure was supposed to be.

How did I get myself into it?

It was saying yes to opportunities

and not shutting myself completely down. It was saying, "Life still may be good. I just have to keep a little slice of my heart open to what's out there."

After I went rock climbing up in New Hampshire, I moved out to Arizona. I got a job as a teacher at this really wonderful school called The Phoenix Country Day School. I joined the Arizona mountaineering club. Outside of Phoenix are all kinds of different geological rock formations.

Pat: Did this start to translate into mountains as you got into mountain climbing or is that a totally different skill set?

Erik: There's overlap, but they're almost like separate disciplines.

I did not gradually work my way into the big mountains. I was climbing a rock base outside of Phoenix with my friend Sam. Sam had attention deficit disorder.

We connected on a challenge. We both had these challenges and that is a great connection point, believe it or not. I got to the top, pulled Sam up, and he said, "We should try something bigger."

I said, "What, like a bigger rock base around here?"

And he goes, no, "Let's try Denali."

And I thought that's totally different. That's not rock climbing in the desert! That's a gigantic 20,300-foot glaciated, freezing- cold mountain in Alaska.

And I hadn't camped out in the snow since I had been a boy scout in eighth grade. So, it was quite a leap into the big mountains.

One of my secrets to success is being impressionable.

And so, when Sam had this grand idea, I said, "Wow, really, you think I can do that? Cool."

We started training, and a year and a half later, after nineteen days of climbing, we summited Denali on Helen Keller's birthday. We didn't know it was her birthday until we got down.

It was really cool. And by the way, we failed on every mountain we tried until we got to Denali.

I started climbing peaks that were off the map, that nobody's really heard of. We'd have climbs where we'd leave at two in the morning and we wouldn't get back down until the next night at 10:00.

I was climbing with one friend of mine who had attempted Everest twice without supplemental oxygen, and he said, "Look, dude, you're better than 90 percent of the people who try Everest."

He pointed out that a lot of the people who try Everest aren't real mountaineers, they're kind of hobby, part-time mountaineers or people that want that mountain on their resume.

He went on to say, "You've dedicated your life to this. You have every right, every chance to be there. You've earned your right to at least give it a try."

And again, being the impressionable person I am, I said okay.

Pat: Did you have any special concerns about Everest versus another mountain?

Erik: For sure, because Everest was way higher than anything I'd ever done. The fear for me was what they call "the death zone." There are varying degrees to the death zone. Some people say it's above 18,000 feet. The extreme death zone is above 26,000 feet.

The altitude and lack of oxygen reduces your brain to a reptilian state.

I rely on my brain so much more than
other people because I can't see.

I'm constantly trying to eke out information from what I'm feeling with my tracking poles or my ice axe or what I'm feeling under my feet. And how steep was this terrain? Was I going to be able to turn around and get down? I was constantly making and calculating in my brain. If I lost that ability, where I couldn't see and I couldn't think, that may be an overwhelming combination.

As it turned out, that was one of my strongest summits. I felt so strong. We got to the summit at 10:00 in the morning, after having left at 9:00 at night, climbing through the dark.

On Everest, we did a lot of things right. It was this combination of Himalaya experience and then blind climbing experience. And that team really, really jelled. In fact, the people on that team have gone on to do great things. Luis Benitez went on to work for the governor; he's head of the outdoor recreation industry in Colorado. Pascalli, PV, our team leader, went on to raft the entire Blue Nile River, which covers thousands of miles from source to sea. Kevin, our base camp manager, went on to guide blind people. I think he got ten blind people to the summit of Kilimanjaro and guided a guy without arms and legs who crabbed his way to the summit of Kilimanjaro.

My team has gone on to do the most amazing things.
And I think it's partly because all our lives were
so transformed by the mountains . . . and everyone
moved on with this yearning to see if they could elevate
other people's lives. Watching what the team did
after the climb has just been magical.

Pat: Pascalli said to you:

Don't let Everest be the greatest thing you ever do.

How do you receive something like that?

Erik: It's one of those things that kind of grows on you. But you've got to realize how thankful I was when I got down alive and safe. PV congratulated the team and pulled me aside.

"Erik, your life's about to change," he said. And he added, " Do me a favor. Don't let this be the greatest thing you ever do."

That was the worst-timed motivational advice in the history of the world.

What PV was saying was that adversity and challenge can shut you down, but success can, too. Those successes can become a trophy on your shelf or a picture on your wall. And he said don't let that happen. He encouraged me to use that accomplishment as energy as a catalyst to propel myself towards new things, towards new areas of growth and ways of connecting and elevating the world in some way. And it took me a while to get what he was saying, but it was so right on.

Pat: You did many things after Everest, but one of them was forming No Barriers. Could you talk a little bit about that?

Erik: Back in the late nineties, I got a call from this guy, Mark Wellman. He was a paraplegic after falling in a climbing accident coming down from a peak in the Sierra Nevada.

He was ice climbing on Mt. Washington, got lost, got frostbite, and lost both legs. He started tinkering in his garage and built these prosthetic legs and feet. Nobody had ever seen anything like it.

Using little rubber wedges of feet to wedge into little seams and cracks, he became an extraordinary climber after losing his legs. And so Mark, Hugh Herr, who's another legend in the climbing world who lost both legs in a climbing accident on ice, and I climbed this tower outside of Moab. It is called Ancient Art and it's this crazy little corkscrew of a summit.

When we got to the top of that climb Mark said, "Not bad for three gimps."

I had never heard that word before. I didn't even know what a gimp was, but Mark kind of uses it as a badge of pride.

It was that climb that was the conception of No Barriers, because I looked at these two guys and I asked, "What's the universal takeaway here?"

There was this great lesson around pioneering and engineering. There was a great lesson around how they took crap and turned it into gold. They took bad things, totally spun them on their head, and made them into these powerful forces.

There were rock towers that were all around us that had been sculpted by the elements into these super beautiful profound structures.

I guess the lesson was you choose how the elements shape you.

Out of that came No Barriers.

I think No Barriers, on a bigger scale, is an antidote for all the challenges and division we're facing as a country.

It's all about leaning in and saying, let's tap into that light that exists within us, the human spirit or whatever you want to call it.

And let's find purpose in our lives and let's use it to elevate the world. It doesn't matter what kind of background or ability or challenge you come from.

Pat: I've read your book, *The Adversity Advantage*, and you talk about three categories of people: Quitters, Campers, and Climbers. You say Quitters are maybe 5 percent to 20 percent; Campers, 65 percent to 90 percent; and Climbers are a rare few. And in your corporate work, I think somebody threw out the figure that about 80 percent of people are Campers. First talk about the categories. How do you move somebody from being a camper to a climber?

Erik: Well, that concept is very much intertwined with the No Barriers life and mindset. It's not like this perfect category, as if you're always a Camper. I'm a Camper quite a bit. Sometimes from training I'm so tired, I just go lay on the couch and eat ice cream and that's fine.

We're all kind of drifting between Quitters, Campers, and Climbers all the time. But Quitters, sadly, have a self-destruct mechanism within them. That's tough to work with, but Campers, we found, were really the most interesting group. They are people who start out climbing, as I think we all do.

And then these barriers get in the way. Maybe there's failure when they try something out of the box. Then they get this trauma running through their soul. It prevents them from trying something big again. Or they wake up one day and realize they're not equipped to take things on anymore.

The barriers that they're confronting just keep beating them down and beating them back until the momentum is killed. And then they get shoved to the sidelines. Now they're camping out, they're stagnating, and all that energy is lost to the world. It's such a tragic thing. We found that so many human beings felt like Campers. They felt like they were not fulfilling their purpose on earth.

And Climbers, they're a rare group of people who figured out a way to break through and keep challenging themselves, exploring, and evolving until the day they die. No Barriers is all about taking folks who have been shoved to the sidelines, camping and starting to stagnate, but they know in their heart that they're not reaching what their potential is.

We get a lot of injured veterans and a lot of people with physical challenges and a lot of people who suffer from fear and anxiety. Kids in the foster care program, first generation Americans. People who struggle with all kinds of things and they say, "Hey, I want to be a Climber, but I just don't quite know how to get there."

What I tell people is:

No Barriers is simply the catalyst, the change comes from them. The motivation comes from them.

We're just an energy or a catalyst to give you some new techniques and ideas to shape a new mindset and a map to go forward and navigate your life.

Pat: A slight change of topic, but I am absolutely fascinated by your kayaking experience, which was not very easy for you, was it?

Erik: No. If I thought climbing was hard, kayaking was like ten times harder because things are happening so fast.

Pat: I have a quote from your book I want to read. You write that:

Climbing was more about bringing yourself forth, asserting your will over an extreme inhospitable environment, yet trying to apply that learning to rivers had failed. Perhaps the secrets of a river were not revealed by trying to exert ego over it, but rather by letting go and in that letting go . . . maybe this was as close as we could ever get to understanding just a brief mortal flash of that light connecting with something bigger, something mysterious and something infinite.

Erik: It was a great life lesson for me. I didn't realize I was a control freak until I started kayaking and realized that there's very little you can control. Going into these rapids, you have to ride that energy and use it. But you cannot fight the river. You're going at the river's pace and the river dictates. And that was hard for me because in climbing you could stop. You can't do that with kayaking. There was no break.

I trained for so many years to kayak the Grand Canyon. I probably trained for eight years.

There were these brief moments between the fear when time slows down. I would go into a rapid like Upset, which is a huge rapid on the Colorado River in the Grand Canyon. I had to hammer left into this wall of water, and then to my right was this gigantic hole that you do not want to go into. That's why they call it Upset. And you're riding this gauntlet between the two.

As you're connecting with this river, you're no longer this entity that's separate from the river and the water. There's no separation between you and the canyon. These moments are brief, like seconds. But that's what they call the flow state.

It's where finally your brain lets go and that separation between you and the experience dissolves.

I sat on the side of the river when I got to camp, in the sunshine by myself, just thinking, that's a spiritual experience. It's this flash of something beyond what we know. Something that the edges of your fingertips are grasping and it's something beautiful and eternal and powerful. And I think you try to seek it out again and again.

Maybe that's the addiction of doing these extreme things; not the idea of defined death, but that brief connection with that mysterious eternity of life.

Thoughts For You to Ponder

How do you feel around someone with a disability? Why? What does it say about you?

Where in your life are you a Quitter, a Camper, or a Climber?

Have you ever had a "flash of something beyond what we know?" Relive it, tell the story, and feel it. What do you feel?

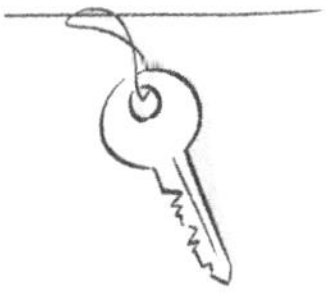

Key Takeaways

- Sometimes you must make the difficult decision to just leave the past behind
- What's within you that is stronger than what's in your way
- You can take "bad" things and turn them into gold

CHAPTER NINE

Trading in the Trading Floor

"With crisis, we either break down or break through."

–TOM CRONIN

Some events break us. But I like to think that we come back stronger, much like the Japanese art of Kintsugi. Kintsugi is the art of putting shattered pottery pieces back together with gold filling the fractures. The idea is that by highlighting the scars, we create something more beautiful and resilient than the original piece.

I especially relate to this ancient art. My imperfections are many. I've been broken several times. But I've come to love my scars because I have become strong. Resilient.

Hitting that breaking point seems to be a very human habit. We stay with what we know until it is no longer possible to do so. And then change must follow. Both Tom Cronin and I had to hit a breaking point in our lives that sent each of us on a quest for peace. And on the other side, we both hit gold.

Reno/Tahoe, 2013

My quest for peace was not very peaceful.

On the one hand, my "incurable but hopefully manageable" cancer that I had been diagnosed with in 2009 had returned (again), and I was told to prepare for a stem cell transplant, a procedure with a 30 percent mortality rate, plus issues of possible rejection and long-term complications.

On the other hand, there were my neighbors-from-hell who had just built a 9,000-square-foot house right on the property line. Their stereo boomed constantly. It was so loud that the windows in my family room flexed back and forth, in and out, expanding and contracting with the beats of the heavy percussion that pounded anything in its path.

My home had become unlivable and my backyard a construction zone as I attempted to block out the neighbors-from-hell by relandscaping my property. A stone wall was built. Semi-mature trees were hauled in and planted. But their stereo kept blasting away. Doom, doom, doom! The base reverberated throughout the entire neighborhood and through my very bones.

One night, against the booming of the bass, I stood amidst the rubble of my yard and looked skyward as if the stars might hold an answer. I was dealing with a recurrent cancer, with a potential transplant, with life and death. And my one place of refuge, my privacy, and my sanity were under relentless attack.

An abyss of pain welled up from my heart into my throat. I looked up at the night sky, and a deep howl rose arose from somewhere within me. I let loose a blood-curdling scream. I screamed again and again and again, a guttural scream of rage, of fear, and of death. And the sound of my pain was drowned by the relentless doom, doom, doom of the stereo next door.

In the quiet of the night, amidst the pounding bass, my screams were heard by no one.

It was soon after this that I saw an ad for a series of meditation classes at the local museum. Desperate, I signed up. One thing led to another, and I committed to a transcendental meditation practice that included two twenty-minute meditation sessions each day. My sanity hung in the balance, and I clung to that schedule, religiously putting in the time to meditate no matter where I was or what I was doing. At a tennis tournament, I meditated. Before dinner, I meditated. Every morning, I meditated. I was desperate. Meditation seemed like my only lifeline.

I had no expectations, but I quickly found peace and even joy in the quiet of my mind. I learned to observe my thoughts and watch them with detachment. My mantra guided me, and I followed. My mind stilled and the world quieted.

Meditation has been life-changing for me. It has taught me about the wonderful depth and blissful solitude of silence. It has taught me about finding space in the moment. It stilled that guttural scream of isolation and pain that started me on this course, and it connected me to an awareness much greater than myself. In the absence of thought, I was able to observe my thoughts. Meditation started to change my orientation from outside myself to within. It dared me to find and experience a truth not tied to the material world.

Meditation is a game changer, and not just for me. For Tom Cronin, it led him from the mania of the bond trading floor and all the alcohol and drugs that went with that lifestyle to a new way of doing business. And it eventually led him to a new business of writing, film production, and teaching. His goal: To get one billion people to meditate.

My Guest, Tom Cronin: Bond Trader, Meditation Guru, Film Producer

Tom Cronin started his professional life as a bond trader.

If anyone has seen Wolf of Wall Street, you'll get a very clear view of what my life was like. . . fast and furious and crazy times!

But the pace of the frantic, alcohol- and drug-riddled lifestyle wasn't sustainable. Tom found himself depressed and on suicide watch.

Then he discovered meditation and this hard charging, high living, bond trader's life changed as he found a profound peace in stillness. Meditation answered a yearning and a doorway to wisdom that had been missing in Tom's life.

His manner of doing business changed. Rather than taking clients drinking, he arranged opera tickets and surfing safaris. And along the way he pondered how he could turn the many lessons he'd learned from the power of meditation into a self-sustaining business.

Tom stayed in the financial business another sixteen years before he took off on his own, with a goal of inspiring one billion people to meditate daily.

Film was one of the avenues he chose to reach a global audience. Although he'd never produced a film, Tom teamed up with Jacqui Fifer to create *The Portal*. The film and book of the same name are a tour de force, integrating the stories of six people who overcame enormous adversity using stillness, meditation, and mindfulness, and expanded their consciousness.

Today, Tom is a coach, meditation teacher, author, and speaker. His goal: Changing the world, one mind at a time, using meditation to do so.

Tom Cronin: The Conversation

This conversation has been edited, but there's so much more to the story! When you have time, scan the QR code and you can listen to the original unedited conversation and view videos and photos of each guest. Or just visit BumpInTheRoad.us/Readers-Portal/ and sign in.

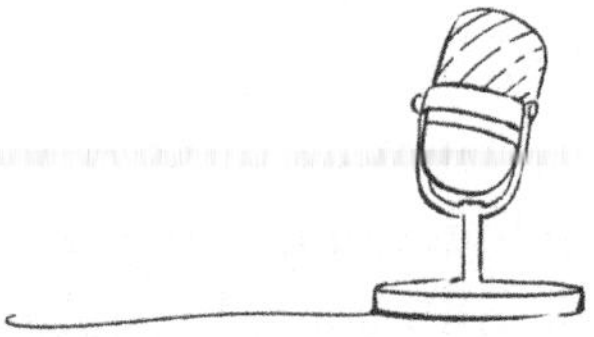

Tom: Today I'm a meditation teacher, speaker, corporate facilitator, and I run retreats. And I was the film producer of *The Portal* film and the writer of *The Portal* book.

My life took quite a turn many years ago, when I was working in finance as a broker on a very hectic trading room floor.

If anyone saw *The Wolf of Wall Street*, you'll get a very clear idea about what my life was like. I started my career as a broker in 1987. They were fast, furious, and crazy times. It was all very good and exciting. I was young and I got swept along by the culture of the late eighties, early nineties finance industry, which included lots of drinking, lots of drugs, and no HR departments. It was very unchecked.

There was glamor and glitz, but over time, I started to have anxiety and panic attacks. Eventually that morphed into a deep, dark depression.

It definitely wasn't the path that I ever imagined myself to be on. I wanted to be a journalist writing articles for *Time* magazine about capitalistic greed. And here I was, a drug-taking broker in the finance industry, earning nearly a million dollars a year. I'd detoured a long way from my orbit without realizing it.

Eventually, I had a full-blown nervous breakdown at the age of twenty-nine. I was put on suicide watch. I was seeing psychiatrists and doctors and psychologists and put on pharmaceutical drugs. I was very lost and didn't really have a sense of identity.

And then that's when I found meditation. It was a fascinating process to discover this thing that was completely alien in my life. It just was like this incredible shift, this sort of illumination that just started to happen. I realized that this was the thing that I'd been looking for all my life.

What I found through the meditation was that connection to something, much purer, much deeper within.

That was the starting point for my journey to get to here.

Pat: Meditation's so interesting. Some people still think it's a little bit woo-woo. And there are so many different types of meditation. I think there's something for everybody. How did you pursue your meditation practice?

Tom: I did a lot of research. There are many different techniques and it's about finding the technique that resonates with you and the one that you can implement and integrate into your day on a daily basis.

When I looked for meditation, I looked for something that would be quite impactful, quite quickly. For me, at the time, it was Transcendental Meditation that put me into a deep state quickly.

Pat: You stayed in finance for sixteen more years. What was it like to manage this loss of identity and reintegrate back into your same job?

Tom: In all transparency, it was very difficult initially because I quickly went from being one of the wildest party guys that was leading the pack to not wanting to do that at all.

Once I started learning to meditate, all those addictions and cravings just melted away and I had to find a way to integrate into this new way of living. Initially, it was very alienating and quite challenging,

but what I learned over time was to really live my truth and do what was true for me.

Part of my job was to entertain clients. These were the bankers and the traders that were dealing lots of money through our company and through me. Developing those relationships usually involved late nights of drinking and nightclubs and parties. But what I found was a new way of doing that. I'd take them and their wives and my wife out for dinner or to the opera or to yoga retreats. We'd go on surfing safaris. And what started to happen was:

I found a way to elevate their life, not deteriorate or detract from their life.

It was great for my business. It really helped because it was a way to add value to my clients' lives.

Pat: That's brilliant.

Tom: Yeah. It was very unique for the industry, I must admit. But I just had to find a way that was going to make it work.

Pat: What made you ultimately decide to leave trading?

Tom: It was just this deep arising that came from within. It just got harder and harder to turn up each day and quote a quarter point movement on a ten-year bond and try and make some money out of that.

Pat: Where did the idea of *The Portal*, both the book and the movie, come from?

Tom: Well, I'd say *The Secret. The Secret* blew me away. They managed to take a film, a book, and a very esoteric subject manner, and they mainstreamed it. The possibility of mainstreaming meditation through a film and book was very exciting to me.

Pat: Tell people a little bit about the project, because it is an astonishingly beautiful and very aggressive project.

Tom: It's been blood, sweat, and tears and I'm still recovering from it. It's been a long nine-year journey.

It was much, much more difficult than I thought and still has its challenges. Trying to get a film out to the world and get people to watch it is a lot more challenging than I thought. I had this idea that it would just go viral, and everyone would watch it and it would become a global phenomenon. Why wouldn't you?

We wanted this film to be something that had an emotional arc that followed the hero's journey. It was quite challenging because we've got six stories that cover global crisis themes.

Each person had a crisis and all of them found that that crisis was a major turning point in their life for evolution.

With crisis only two things can happen.
We either break down or break through.

So, we want to make sure as a species that we break through to a new way of living. And

that requires opening our minds, connecting to our hearts, and discovering what's deep within us.

Thoughts For You to Ponder

Have you ever made a change that isolated you from your social tribe?

Have you ever broken down? How did you break through?

What personal strength helped you move forward? (If you're curious, ViaCharacter.org provides a fascinating look at your personal strengths with the idea of helping you navigate your best life.)

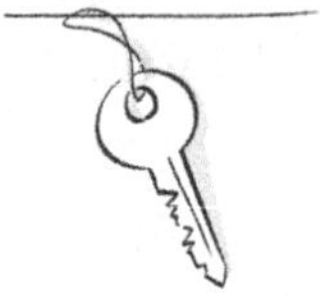

Key Takeaways

- The status quo is not the only way to do things
- Find your truth and live it
- It's in stillness that we experience consciousness

CHAPTER TEN

Yes is Where the Fun Is

"It's good to see you."

–NICK ADKINS

Nick Adkins would say, "Yes is where all the fun is." Saying yes opens doors. Saying yes leads to adventure. Saying yes is about connecting with life.

But these days, as we swim in a sea of connectivity, do we really connect with life? Or are we connecting with an illusion? How often do we scan our devices, pushing buttons, our minds in a faraway imaginary world rather than in the conversation at hand? How often do we half listen, and half understand?

Being present and truly seeing another person is becoming something of a lost art. Being seen is a fundamental need for all of us. It answers our very human need to engage and to matter. Instead, we are captivated by the trivial and the bauble du jour. We share images and gossip via our devices, caught up in the false reflections of others. And we wonder why we feel lost and disconnected!

Sometimes I wonder if it's the lack of inner reflection that renders us susceptible to these imaginary worlds. Without inner reflection, we cannot connect with ourselves. And if we can't connect with ourselves, how can we possibly find something in common with others?

In this chapter, two very different people take two very different routes to connecting, both with themselves and with the world at large. In my case, I hit the road again. And in Nick's case, hitting the road to Burning Man and saying yes to the simple act of giving and receiving upends his life in ways he never could have expected.

Reno/Tahoe, 2015

I had moved from Lake Tahoe down to the Sierra foothills at the base of Mt. Rose. From my family room window, I could watch the snow cats groom the ski slopes. It was twenty minutes and a few thousand feet of elevation from my driveway to the lift line.

I had created my perfect house, with a massive library, rare maps on the walls, and an organic garden in the yard. A trellis was covered with purple wisteria, and underneath an off-white Brazilian hammock moved lazily in the breeze. This house helped me to express the beauty I felt in my soul.

I think I have always felt that beauty, but recent life events had focused me on the wonder of it all. I had just navigated six years of on-again/off-again cancer treatment. It had changed the way I view life. It had changed me.

The biggest change came in an intense desire to share what I had learned, to give back, and to help others avoid the terrible isolation that I had experienced, particularly with cancer.

I created a tech platform that addressed these issues and so much more. It was about compassion and connection, especially through long-term illness. To pitch this platform to Silicon Valley investors, I needed a beta version that would provide the metrics needed to assess my idea.

But I don't code.

So, I hired a group that did.

And I waited. And waited. Time passed. Too much time. I called, I emailed. There was no response.

The tech group never did deliver my platform. But they did take all my intellectual property and register it with the U.S. Patent Office as their own. According to my very expensive lawyers, a lawsuit was my only option. It would cost *in increments* of half a million dollars, take three years of my life, and there was no guaranteed outcome.

Seriously?

I was sick on so many levels. I had poured my hard-earned, heart-felt, soulful best into that project. I was depending on it to monetize a website that I'd built around the cancer experience. I had the audience; I understood the market. I just needed some data to bring in the investment.

My hair started to fall out again (from stress, not chemo) and I was vomiting blood. My oncologist assured me that he could find something wrong with me. And of course, the elephant in the room was that the lymphoma had recurred, yet again.

A host of expensive and invasive medical tests loomed. The lawyers demanded more money even as the tech group refused to engage. They simply waited for a lawsuit they knew I couldn't afford.

I had had it.

Six years of chemo, radiation, and surgery and all the financial, emotional, and existential stress that goes with it. Six years of my life where sometimes the chemo worked for a while and sometimes it didn't. Six years of having my life turned totally upside down. I simply couldn't do it again.

If the past was indicative of the future, I figured I had eighteen to twenty-four months before the cancer overran my body yet again. I had weathered tumors that wrapped around my aorta, spread throughout my body, and threatened my brain. I had battled the medical establishment to get the care I needed and became my own advocate to avoid the potentially deadly medical mistakes that loomed at every decision point. I had endured almost unbearable isolation. I simply couldn't go through it all again.

The legal bills grew. Medical bills mounted. I had no support and I saw no future. Goodness knows events had toughened me, but I didn't know if even I was tough enough to face this.

The vague malaise I had felt months before manifested itself in a desire to simply rid myself of baggage. I wanted to rid myself of the baggage of cancer, of illness, of a long-ago ex, of too much stuff. I hadn't thought through what I was actually seeking; I just knew I had to simplify my life. Somehow.

I've always had a saying: "When the going gets tough, the tough go traveling."

Perhaps it's running away. Perhaps it's a period of reflection. Travel for me is both a mirror and a balm. It's a reminder of happy childhood times. It's a space of possibility. Once again, the road beckoned me forward and I said yes to whatever this next chapter might hold.

I sold my house, the wonderful haven I had created, and put my carefully selected and curated belongings in storage. My rare map collection was packed away. My aviation books, my history books, and my cookbooks were put into boxes. Each represented a vital part of me. Were they some sort of discarded sum of my life, destined indefinitely for storage? And what did that mean for me?

"Oh, you're going traveling," people would respond.

There seemed to be no comprehension of what I had been through or the utter uncertainty I was facing. As always, I put a good face on it all and managed everything with impeccable capability. I was left with the distinct impression that no one, absolutely no one, saw me. I was utterly on my own.

The house sold quickly. I had no idea where I was heading or how long my health would hold. I simply headed west, just as I had years ago with Whiskey Oscar. Only this time I was traveling alone. From California, I went north to Canada, to Europe, South America, and to Africa.

As I traveled, I wrote. I sought answers about betrayal, trust, and life. In looking within, perhaps for the first time in my life, I saw me. I saw this curious, creative, giving person with all her foibles. I saw her strengths, weaknesses, and insecurities. I liked this person. This was someone I could really spend time with. And it finally dawned on me: I was really the only person who needed to see me.

And with that realization, I started seeing others.

Meet My Guest, Nick Adkins: Healthcare Executive, Entrepreneur

"I see you," Nick says as he greets people.

His direct gaze and kindness are immediately evident.

Nick Adkins cuts a striking figure with his long beard, kilt, and PinkSocks. It's a far cry from his corporate days of suits and ties. But then, so is his mission for kindness.

Nick is the co-founder of PinkSocks, a movement about creating a global community of empathy, community, and love. PinkSocks are tall, pink socks with black mustaches printed into the fabric. Their quirkiness is a curiosity and they open the door to many a conversation.

PinkSocks is a phenomenon that had no design or plan to become that. It was simply born out of the ethos of giving.

The giving ethos has its roots in Nick's first trip in 2010 to Burning Man. Burning Man is a community and temporary city of over 70,000 people that is created by Burners (the attendees) in the Nevada desert each year. It's an event focused on community, art, self-expression, and self-reliance.

There are ten principles of Burning Man. Gifting was the principle that captured Nick's imagination.

The principle of gifting does not require quid pro quo.

If you give me something, I don't have to give you a gift in return.

A person's accepting the other's gift IS the gift. Accepting with gratitude and love. Seeing, really seeing, the other person in that moment . . . that's the magic!

And Nick has found a way to bring that magic into the every day. This is his story.

Nick Adkins: The Conversation

This conversation has been edited, but there's so much more to the story! When you have time, scan the QR code and you can listen to the original unedited conversation and view videos and photos of each guest. Or just visit BumpInTheRoad.us/Readers-Portal/ and sign in.

Pat: PinkSocks is such a story of transformation on a personal and global level. Would you tell our listeners a little bit about PinkSocks and how it came to be?

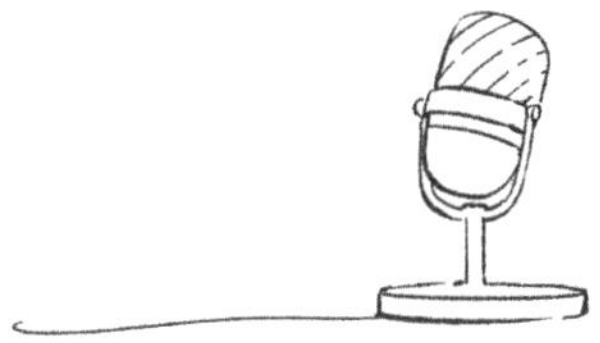

Nick: PinkSocks is really a movement; a phenomenon that had no design or no plan to become that.

It was simply born out of this ethos of gifting.

I was a co-founder of a health tech startup in Portland, Oregon. Co-founder and CTO Andrew Richards and I went to a healthcare conference in Chicago in 2015. We thought it would be fun to load up our backpacks with these pink socks with black mustaches on them and give those away at the conference. And that's what we did. Every time someone would come up and say, "Hey, what's the story with those socks?" it was an opportunity for us to connect with someone and say, "Hey, I'm Nick, I'm Andrew, what's your name? What's your story?"

I didn't think of anything beyond that. We did it for a year. It was great. We met a lot of people and made a lot of new friends. About that time, someone reached out to me on Twitter and asked if we sent some pink socks to somebody in the Netherlands. And I was like, "No, why?"

He said, "Well, there's a guy over there who has sourced PinkSocks and is gifting PinkSocks in the Netherlands to help drive awareness for the work that he's doing with Alzheimer's and dementia care."

Someone sent me another message that said, "Did you send PinkSocks to somebody in Wales? There's a guy in Wales who's gifting PinkSocks to help drive awareness for the work they he's doing with ataxia, a rare disease."

It was at that moment that we realized that PinkSocks had gone organic and global.

I got invited to do a TEDx talk in San Francisco in 2017, and PinkSocks has just taken off. We've gifted PinkSocks to over 100,000 people all around the world. I'm grateful to be a part of it. It's fun to watch every day.

Pat: Well gifting is fun and PinkSocks is gifting with the purpose of connection. I think true connection is unfortunately much rarer than we think in this world.

Nick: You would think we would be super-connected.

There's a difference between connectivity and connection.

The world is swimming in connectivity. But we rarely look up from our phones. We rarely take our earbuds out.

We don't want to confuse connectivity with connection. They're different things. And what the PinkSocks allow you to do is have an authentic connection with another person. Just like on the back of the label of the PinkSocks, it says:

Every time you wear your PinkSocks, you're going to connect with someone new.

Don't miss each one of those moments. When you wear your PinkSocks, someone comments and says, "I like those, those are cool, those are fun, those are funky, what's the story?"

Boom, that's the universe right there, tapping you on the shoulder saying, "Okay here it is. Take your earbuds off, get off your phones, stay on the train another stop and introduce yourself and say, 'I'm Pat, what's your name?'"

It's in those beautiful moments of connection of one on one where the magic really happens, where we're able to practice some empathy and see the humanity in each other. And it never gets old.

When I meet people, I never say it's good to meet you. I say:

It's good to see you.

There's different energy around those phrases. Being seen is so important for all of us as humans. It's this craving for connection that we all have, that's hardwired into our DNA. We all want it as humans.

Pat: PinkSocks grew out of your experience at Burning Man.

Nick: I went to Burning Man for my first time in 2010. At that time, I was a suit and tie COO of a healthcare company in Nashville, Tennessee.

Burning Man always occurs at the same time each year. It's the week before Labor Day. I'd already bought tickets. I prefaced the decision with, depending on where my dad is, I may be able to go, or I may not be able to go. My father had chronic lymphocytic leukemia. He died on June 10, 2010. When he passed, it gave me the permission I needed to go to desert that year in late August.

I went with no expectations. In a video I caught late one night before I left, the narrator said, "You've all been studying, you're so ready. You've got the 10 Burning Man principles. In fact, some of you have probably got things into a spreadsheet. Now what you have to do is just come to the desert and let go of all of that, let go of all the expectations, just show up, just be open, willing, and present to have an experience."

So that's what I did. I put myself in a space where I was going to say yes, and I was going to let go of a lot of conditioning of fear and constructs of judgment and just see how beautiful it could feel. I've been back several times now, and each time it's just such a wonderful experience.

And what a change that has made in my life. What if we could apply the principles of Burning Man in our everyday life? What a magical place the world could be!

I came home from that first Burning Man in 2010, and we were trying to decide what to do with the company at that time. A lot of things were rolling out in healthcare. Should we sell the company now? Should we merge with another company? Should we acquire another company? Should we take on some more debt? What was the best strategy?

The Board asked, "What's your vote on the company?"

I said, "Sell it. I'm done."

"What are you going to do?"

"I'm going to move to Portland, Oregon, and become a hippie."

At that time, I was forty-five years old. I came to realize that life is not linear. It's not on this zero-to-eighty-year timeline. It's spiraling in and out all the time. It's not a series of 'if, then' equations.

We're all one phone call away from 'you've got cancer.' We're all one heartbeat away from a heart attack or a stroke. There is no guarantee of the 'if, then' equation being solved. Life's happening right now in every moment, don't miss it. And that's a philosophy that I adopted as soon as I got back.

I'm going to live every day like it's my last day. I'm going to wake up grateful.

I've been doing that now for the last eleven years and practicing it every day. It's made a difference for me.

Pat: You bring up two themes that have come out of *Bump in the Road* with some of my other guests. One that life is not linear. And just say yes.

Nick: I start my Ted talk with the word. Yes.

"Yes" is where the fun is. "Yes" is where the adventure is. If you say no, the story ends.

And so it is. And the universe, it's so vast. Life's so majestic and beautiful and wonderful. And that goes on and on and on beyond this limited life that we may experience here on Earth. It's just a moment against the backdrop of the expanse of the universe.

Why say no to so much stuff? And the answer is because we're conditioned with fear. We've grown up with it. The media, everything, it's just fear, and more fear. One of two things are going to drive every bit of our lives, and that's love or fear. You're going to make a choice. They always coexist. And we must choose which one we want to focus on.

The small things *are* the big things. The cumulative effect of the small things is what changes the world. I tell people, "Please, social media is not good for you. Just get off of it. Don't look at it, because there's so much of it is just fear. Stop watching TV, stop watching the news."

Follow what your heart knows to be true.

Your heart knows that people are inherently good. See yourself in the other person, see your brother, your sister, your mom, your father, your son, your daughter, we're so similar.

PinkSocks is a good opportunity to practice empathy and joy.

One of the things I've come to know about empathy is that we want to fix a problem. We want to make it better. We want to make it go away.

Well, so many times our job isn't to fix it, isn't to make it go away, but it's to bear witness to it, to share space with the pain, to share space with the hurt and the fear, the sadness that our friends and others are going through, to just let the process unfold, let the path have its journey. It's a practice, because we all want to help people. So, we ask ourselves what we can do to help. Sometimes the realization is that you can't do anything.

Pat: But you can show up. And that means a lot.

Nick: Just to bear witness, to share space with it, and say, "I see you. I love you. I see the pain you're going through. I see the hurt. I see that. I see you."

Pat: If you could leave people with a few words of wisdom or advice in terms of living a PinkSocks life, what would you say to them?

Nick: Love more. Just love more.

Thoughts For You to Ponder

Are you "seen?" Do you give others the chance to be "seen?"

Practice empathy and joy this week. Notice how you feel. Notice the impact you have on those around you.

How could you love more?

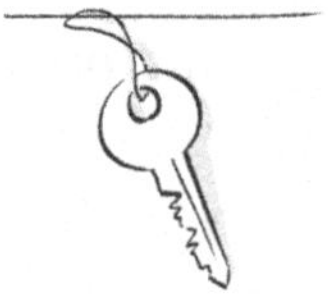

Key Takeaways

- We all need to be seen
- Connectivity is not connection
- Just say yes; yes is where the fun is

CHAPTER ELEVEN

Gratitude–It's in My Genes

"I would also say this is a such a great life."

–EFFIE PARKS

Gratitude is profound. A gratitude practice can shift your life from a glass half empty to a glass half full. It's a chance to tell your story in a way that benefits you.

This chapter is about having the courage to change your perception in order to change your world. It's a story of finding gratitude in the most unexpected places. Ultimately, it's a story of letting go of what was "supposed to be," of surrendering, and finding gratitude for what is.

Reno/Tahoe, Nevada, 2009-2015

Cancer has been the most isolating experience of my life. Yet it introduced me to gratitude in a way I had not previously understood.

I first had a gratitude practice after my divorce. I would sit in my bed, which was a mattress on a metal frame. The room was bare and there was one lamp with one light bulb for the whole room. Every morning, I'd force myself to find just one thing to be grateful for. Many days, it was a challenge that eluded me.

Gratitude reappeared in my life in a powerful way with cancer. It made me realize that each moment was precious, and I was so very grateful for the smallest things. Beauty was everywhere. A hummingbird poised mid-air by the wisteria; the warmth of the spring sun on my back in the swaying hammock; the sunrise as it spread down the eastern side of the Sierra. It made me aware that each moment had to count because no one is guaranteed another.

While I may have discovered the power of gratitude, life was far from perfect. I was extremely isolated. Friends dropped away. A five-year relationship couldn't survive the deep spiritual and emotional questions I faced. My world was re-arranging itself, without my permission. I could do nothing but surrender to the isolation, the uncertainty, and time. Time. What is time and how much did I have? I had no control over anything.

With the isolation I experienced, I craved connection. This experience isn't unique to cancer. It's often present in the day-to-day when we don't feel that we fit in. Maybe you're the clumsy one in yoga, or the less than popular one in your group, or the chubby one in the land of the thin. We all feel isolation and seek connection.

But connection isn't always there when we most want or need it. It seldom shows up on our terms. When all else fails, I have learned to be still. To surrender. Because in surrender, there is gratitude for what is. And when we let go of what isn't "right" and see the beauty before us, in people, in nature, and in ourselves, our perceptions shift, and a new path emerges.

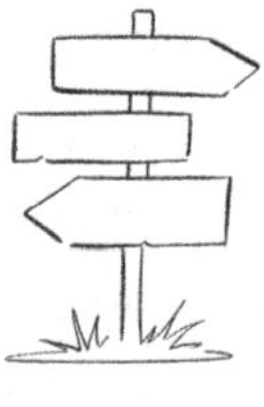

Meet My Guest, Effie Parks: Podcaster, Parent

Dreams of a perfect childhood, a perfect child, and the perfect life are part of every soon-to-be mother's wish list. Effie Parks did find the perfect child, but it took her on a path she never expected.

I had these fictional ideas of what my
life was going to be like as a mom.

Effie's child Ford was born disabled, with an extremely a rare disease called CTNNB1 syndrome, a cell growth neurological disorder. As a result, Ford has several disabilities. He needs a wheelchair, has no verbal skills, and suffers from a combination of low trunk tone and dystonia in his arms and legs. The disease, CTNNB1 syndrome, was discovered in 2012 and worldwide, there were only fifty cases when Ford was diagnosed.

Motherhood can be isolating for anyone, but the shock, the magnitude, and the isolation that went with Ford's birth and disability were overwhelming.

So, Effie started *Once Upon a Gene*, a podcast that would connect her with a worldwide audience of parents, disabled children, and their siblings. The podcast connects families and individuals trying to find their way in a disabled world; a world that most of the rest of us know nothing about.

My podcast came about out of desperation. I was so isolated,
so sad, so lost. I knew there had to be other people like me.

Dealing with disability, in Effie's life, involves juggling work, giving Ford injections, connecting with scientists, trying to have a social life, and keeping tabs on her own mental health. It's a complex and ever-changing set of demands.

How has it changed me? I honestly couldn't list the ways.
You just really learn what's important.
It just slows things down in a really good way.

Ford's disability has impacted the whole family. Effie notes that in addition to turning her world upside down, it has inspired Ford's sister to develop a highly-tuned emotional IQ. The impact of having a disabled brother or sister means that siblings quickly recognize what's important in life.

Siblings are one of biggest worries and our biggest treasures. They are the most compassionate, empathetic unsung heroes walking among us.

Life for the Parks family is very different than what they'd imagined. Daily life is a challenge. Effie realized that she could fight this or surrender to it. And when she surrendered, her life changed. Her perspective of disability shifted, and her isolation turned to connection, both for herself and for others. In this podcast, I ask Effie if she could rewrite her story, would she? Her answer will leave you breathless.

Effie Parks: The Conversation

This conversation has been edited, but there's so much more to the story! When you have time, scan the QR code and you can listen to the original unedited conversation and view videos and photos of each guest. Or just visit BumpInTheRoad.us/Readers-Portal/ and sign in.

Effie: My podcast came about from desperation and because it didn't exist. I found myself in a place where I couldn't go on that way anymore. I was so isolated so sad, and so lost. I knew there had to be other people out there like me. I had to find them because I didn't like feeling like that. And that wasn't who I was.

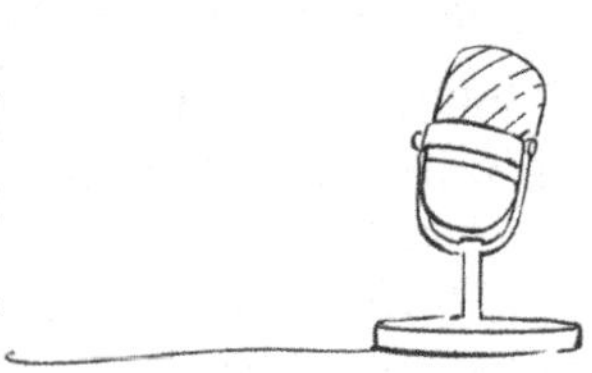

I looked for this community and I couldn't find it. I kind of found little bits and pieces, and that gave me hope that I could help someone like me not feel as crummy as I was feeling.

At one point I just Googled: how do I make a podcast? That was the beginning. And the second I started, the energy, the intention, everything that I knew needed to be there came together.

Pat: Now what spurred the search for this podcast?

Effie: Five years ago, I gave birth to my very first kiddo. His name's Ford and he was born with a rare genetic disease called CTNNB1 syndrome. So rare. It's just named by the gene at this point.

When he was born, that isn't something I expected in the slightest.

I had these fictional ideas of what my life was going to be like as a mom . . . and who my kid was going to be, and all the things that we were going to experience together. And then that was demolished, and we were told, "We don't know anything about the disease. Go home and love your kid."

That was an introduction to motherhood that was not even remotely on my radar.

Pat: What symptoms does your son have?

Effie: This gene prevents him from producing enough of a protein called beta catenin. This is a very important protein for cell growth, cell health, cell reproduction, and cell adhesion. It's a neurological disorder. He can't sit or crawl or walk. He uses a wheelchair for his independence and mobility. He is non-verbal. He cannot speak. He has very low tone in his trunk area, which prevents him from swallowing and clearing mucus from his chest. So, he uses a G-tube to be fed. He has severe dystonia in his arms and legs, so he doesn't have the best control over them.

There are several other weird things, like he has sparse white hair and white skin. He has microcephaly, which is a very small head. He has a bunch of random little things like that, that come along with the genetic abnormality. We don't know a lot about it yet. We're in the beginning stages.

It was discovered in 2012. All the patients are fairly young. There are almost three hundred kids worldwide at this point. There were only fifty when my son was diagnosed.

Pat: I can't imagine what a shock that had to be, particularly in this culture, this kind of super baby pregnancy culture that we find ourselves living in.

Effie: It's funny you say that. There's a book called *Raising a Rare Girl* by Heather Lanier, and she talks about the fact that she was determined to have a super baby.

We're all given this grand idea of don't eat this, don't do this. Everything will be lovely. Everything is perfect. Your kid is going to be popular and fun and do sports and be smart and be an astronaut. You just get enamored with this idea of who you think your kids should be or could be, and how your life is going to look.

You don't really think about the fact that this is all fictional. This is just you *imagining,* but you get so tied to it that when that is abruptly thrown out it is a shock because you really thought it was true. You thought you would get that, because why wouldn't you?

Pat: How has it changed your perspective and how's it changed you?

Effie: I honestly couldn't list the ways and get all of them on this show. I had no idea that this entire population existed. Obviously, I knew there were people with terrible diseases and there were people dying, but it was over there.

People who are disabled are our largest minority. And it seems to be one of the most invisible ones. That blew a giant hole in my house.

How have I not been involved? How have I not noticed?
How have I not helped?

That was huge for me, especially now that I'm raising my own little disabled dude. I have to call ahead everywhere I go to see if I can come. I have to fight all the time to make sure that he can just get in a door somewhere. I have to make sure of so many things that I never imagined and that I didn't know.

Pat: I've often thought that we're all disabled in our own ways, whether it is a perspective we have or a faulty belief system. I think everybody has their things, but I think our society is so hard on people who don't fit the so-called norm.

Effie: It's heartbreaking. I felt so much shame and guilt at first when they told me what my son was going to be like. I was horrified. And I was like, "Oh my gosh, did I do something?"

People talk about it like it's hush-hush or taboo. He is the funniest kid in town and he's amazing. And what he can do is so much more than most adults I know. Why didn't anybody tell me that?

Pat: I think that there is so much more to any of us than what we appear to be. Being disabled, people tend to react poorly to anything that is not within their narrow scope of 'the way things are.' It can be disability, it can be cancer, it can be unemployment. It can be anything that causes them to experience fear. I think it's all fear-based.

Effie: People don't like being uncomfortable.

And a lot of people just don't even have the skills to show up and be empathetic. Not everyone knows how to do that.

Pat: You must live in a constant state of uncertainty. Is there any upside to the uncertainty?

Effie: Yes, perspective.

The upside is I don't worry about the stuff
that other parents are worrying about now.

And I am so grateful for that. I made a joke the other day on my show that this woman on a Facebook group was totally stressing out about what lunchbox to buy for her second grader. It was so important, and this and that. And I was just like, wow. I am so glad I don't have to worry about that. That is so silly.

I've learned how to be in the moment and to savor them.
I know that I don't know what his future looks like.
It just slows things down in a really, really good way.

Pat: I think that these sorts of things deeply challenge our beliefs. And that's never an easy thing to look at. How do you go about channeling this continual uncertainty that you deal with? In addition to being present, what else do you do to cope? How do you take care of yourself?

Effie: First of all, I learned that self-care isn't fancy. It's not pretty. It's not expensive. It's not an event. It's not a trip. It is the little habits that you put into your daily life, no matter what. The non-negotiables.

I have this giant chalkboard magnet on my fridge and I have four oxygen tanks on it. My sister told me to put the four things in each oxygen tank that I must do every single day, no matter what. I put drinking water, breathing practice, eating something healthy, and going outside. Four things, no matter what, I check off my list every single day. Not only do I feel like I accomplish something, especially on the really hard days, but I know those things are sustaining me and giving me life. They're free and I can do them. And I feel proud of myself when I do.

I really try to take care of myself in small ways that I know add up and have a big impact.

I like to wear bright pink, like as much as possible. Most of the time I'm in bright pink or a bright red lipstick. When I see myself in the mirror walking by, it makes me smile. Those things also help me snap back.

But it was connection that changed my life through this podcast.

The people that I've met and the stories that I've heard . . . I get so much out of every single one of them. And then I see this chain reaction of connection and care that happens every single time. And that fills me up.

Pat: Ford has siblings, yes?

Effie: Yes. Ford has a two-year-old little sister.

Pat: How do they get along?

Effie: They get along great. Ford is really enamored with her. He loves watching her and he loves it when she comes and kisses him goodnight. Izzie is so tender with Ford and it's not because we taught her how to be.

She just knows.

Siblings are one of our biggest worries and our biggest treasures.

They are the most compassionate, empathetic, unsung heroes walking among us.

Most of them go onto careers that contribute to help other people. Izzie's his protector. She's going to educate her friends if they're making fun of Ford or if they're not including him.

She has a gift that these other kids are going to have to learn. This is normal for her.

Pat: She'll grow up with such a richer emotional intelligence than she would have otherwise.

Effie: She already has it.

Pat: Do you think that's common in most siblings?

Effie: Yes. It's a phenomenon we all talk about. They appreciate the small things, and they have a recognition of what's important.

They turn into magnificent human beings.

Pat: The idea that at a young age you develop this hierarchy of what's important or isn't is astonishing. I think it takes adversity for people to start digging deep on an emotional and spiritual level. The positive side of that is the rich rewards you get out of it. But most of us avoid pain. Digging deep is painful.

Effie: Digging deep is painful, but I feel like once you start to do it and you tap into it and you practice it,

it's like a muscle, you get stronger

You learn, you evolve, and while it's painful, you know that if you don't do it, the repercussions are a lot worse.

Pat: What advice would you give to a mother who has a disabled child?

Effie: You have to feel it. You have to let yourself acknowledge all of the feelings that come with it and know that's okay and there's no shame. There's nothing wrong with all the gross icky feelings that you might have. They're human, everyone has them. And if they say they don't, they're not telling the truth.

You go through those stages. You feel angry and sad and betrayed and jealous. Just let those emotions happen, because if you suppress them, they're going to grow and they're going to make you sick.

I would also say that this is a such a great life.

I'm so glad I get to be this person and not the other person that I probably would've been had I had a kid who wasn't like Ford.

Sure, I don't want him to be sick. I don't like the uncertainty, but I think about the Effie that doesn't have this kid. And then I think about the Effie I am now. I am so grateful that this is my life and that this is my awareness. I'm grateful that this is my kid because I've seen him change my entire family. I've seen him change my friends.

I've seen so much magic from it.

And I've become a better person. So just know that there's so much good, even though it's scary and it sucks and it's not fair.

Pat: What plans do you have for *Once Upon a Gene,* your podcast? It's a great name by the way.

Effie: Thank you. Against all podcasting guru advice, I've always just said that I'm going to let this podcast's energy take it wherever it goes. And it has taken me to so many places already.

I've started to do a little series of short interviews on the show once a month. People are just breathtaking. It really does something to people when they get to tell their story or when they get to just be vulnerable.

Pat: You need that emotional connection. And when you have that emotional connection, it's so powerful. It just strips everything else away. It's magical.

Effie:

Especially if you're ready to listen and you're ready to make a change. You can't turn back when things align.

Thoughts For You to Ponder

What are five things you are grateful for? Could you put this into practice each morning at the start of your day?

Have you ever felt 'less than' those around you? Less athletic, less pretty, less smart, less wealthy? How do you react to those feelings? What do you say to yourself?

Think of a problem you are facing. How might things change if you changed your perspective? Could you see your situation through the lens of gratitude?

(Check out the on-line workbook for an exercise on this)

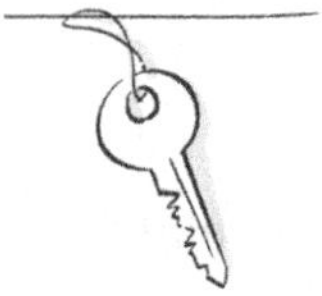

Key Takeaways

- Living a simpler life is powerful
- You must feel whatever it is you're going through
- Be here now

CHAPTER TWELVE

Keep Climbing

"You're not going to conquer that mountain; you're going to conquer yourself."

–SEAN SWARNER

Mountains are one of our greatest metaphors for challenge. And they metaphorically exist in many places. Getting that grade, that new job, or in an athletic feat. We all have our mountain to climb.

But ultimately, attaining any goal is about overcoming our own self-imposed limitations. It's about looking within, dispelling the myths that limit us, and finding courage and strength to take that next step. And the next.

What are the keys to reaching our goals? Where does simple perseverance come into play? Is perseverance really simple? What lessons can we take away from the experience?

Somewhere Outside Philadelphia, 1993

The greenest grass runway in the world nestled into the countryside outside of Philadelphia. It was a summer day, and as the earth warmed, the dew dissipated and clouds formed.

Pilots from around the East Coast had brought their planes and crews to this racing camp, where the skills and knowledge of flying an efficient and fast course would be taught.

At least that was the goal. What evolved for me was something totally different.

We were each assigned to a group. Maps in hand, we discussed the course we'd fly. This was before the days of GPS. Navigation was a critical part of flying. And navigating over unknown terrain, over a countryside of green fields, green crops, and more green fields, while circling in drifting, erratic thermals was not easy.

Maps are rather large, and in the cockpit, refolding and rearranging your map is something of an art. Or a hazard. As we plotted our course, we decided to cut off the extraneous parts of the map to focus on flying and speed. We'd rendezvous in the air and proceed.

Except that the rendezvous in the sky didn't exactly work out. One of the four of us never showed up. Thankfully that wasn't me. Yet.

We set off. Our leader, an experienced competition pilot, rapidly left me in the dust. Learning to fly fast is not easy, and I thought I'd mastered at least some of the art. Apparently not.

It wasn't long before I was on my own and completely lost. I can't explain what it's like to be lost in a strange locale in a sailplane. First you quell the fear and fly the plane. To fly the plane, you must continually be looking for sources of lift. Lift is usually found in rising columns of air called thermals. As you climb in a thermal, you drift with the wind.

Then, you must figure out where you are again, get back on course, and consider where you might find your next source of lift while staying focused on your destination. Sailors tack into the wind to find lift for their sails to generate speed. Sailplane pilots tack into lift to find altitude then trade that altitude for distance and speed.

Navigating on land is relatively forgiving. Navigating on the sea or in the air is not. In the sea, and in the air, when you're lost, you can't pull over on Cloud Nine and ask directions. You are on your own.

That day, the mid-day air had become still. Dead still. I was starting to get nervous. There seemed to be no lift anywhere.

I cruised slowly, nursing every foot of altitude. But no matter what I did, Whiskey Oscar and I were getting lower and lower. The humid mid-Atlantic air was getting warmer and thicker. Sweat soaked through my hat and ran down my brow. The sweat was a combination of the summer heat and my own rising fear. I needed to find a place to land. And soon. Very soon.

Ahead I spied a school with a black roof. And where there's a school, there may be fields. Perhaps a nice big soccer field?

No such luck. Instead, there was a football field with bleachers, goal posts, and a fence. Perhaps it might have been land-able, but not for me, not at my skill level, not at this distance and altitude, and not with the primal fear which rose in my throat as Whiskey Oscar and I got lower and lower.

A black tar roof on the school looked like my only hope. Not for landing (at least I hoped not), but for finding lift. Perhaps, just perhaps, the dark roof had heated up enough to kick off some nice hot rising air and Whiskey Oscar and I could find some altitude.

We came in just a few hundred feet over the roof, banked, and lost about forty-five feet as I entered a tight turn searching for lift. I watched helplessly as the altimeter drifted downward. I literally held my breath as the hand on the altimeter stabilized after that first turn. I was neither climbing nor sinking.

Whiskey Oscar and I circled in place over the black tar roof. I stayed in that turn, around and around, ever so carefully. I flew as slow as I could to maximize any chance of finding lift. If I got too slow, I risked stalling and spinning in. Whiskey Oscar climbed best in a slight slip, but I decided to forgo the slip and be super conservative. I could not afford to stall.

Groups of kids started to gather in the parking lot, pointing and waving. The crowd grew. I turned off my radio and ignored the commotion on the ground to focus on the task at hand.

Patience. I was always impatient and I often mused that I was put on this Earth to learn patience. That day tested my patience, my airmanship, and maybe my life. Ten minutes. Twenty minutes. Thirty. Forty. The cockpit was stifling. The heat and humidity permeated everything. I was soaked in sweat.

From holding the stick so hard and so long, I could hardly move my right hand. An aching discomfort consumed my left arm, which was floating the flaps in just the right position to maximize my climb. Or in that case, my lack of descent.

The only sound was an audio variometer that chirped with a deep sinister tone as the air outside the plane descended, and with a lighter, happier tone as the air rose. After forty minutes of circling, it just emitted a flat, dull groan, indicating neither lift nor sink.

And then I felt it. A slight bump under my right wing. I stayed exactly where I was, silently praying for lift. I didn't dare move away from the promise of that bump of air.

I stared at the altimeter, willing it to climb. Sure enough, it was slowly, oh so slowly, registering a slight increase in altitude. A bubble of hot and rising air had finally kicked off that high school roof. Foot by precious foot, Whiskey Oscar found her pace and we climbed. The crowd in the parking lot below waved goodbye. The variometer chirped happily. Round and round we went, trying to stay centered in that invisible column of rising air until finally my altimeter read 6,000 feet.

For the first time in over an hour, I took a deep breath. I pried my hand off the stick. Altitude was my friend, and I was so deeply grateful for every foot of it. But I was also physically and emotionally spent, and I still had to find the airport I had taken off from and land. It is said that flying is the second greatest thrill known to man. Landing is the first. For the moment, I was grateful to simply have some altitude. I would deal with landing later.

I turned the radio back on and it came alive with half a dozen frantic voices. Other pilots were struggling, too. They called out, asking where I found that lift. I relayed the information about the school roof and watched as several planes, thousands of feet below me, dashed that way in the hope of repeating my minor miracle.

I gave a silent prayer to the Sky Gods; not my fellow pilots but those omniscient and powerful forces of the sky that allowed me to find that little bubble of lift. Whiskey Oscar rewarded me with a happy and buoyant flex of her wings. In the air, she was in her element.

Perseverance, along with some serious luck, saved the day. (Of course, one could argue that I shouldn't have been in that situation at all, but let's forgo that discussion for now.) In the parlance of Sean Swarner, it was time to keep climbing. And climbing, physically, spiritually, and metaphorically, is the essence of Sean Swarner's story.

Meet My Guest, Sean Swarner: Coach, Mountaineer, Explorer

Sean Swarner is a real-life inspiration and a walking example of what is possible.

At the age of thirteen, Sean's life was irreparably changed when he was diagnosed with Hodgkin's lymphoma. He was given three months to live.

And then, a year later, a totally unrelated cancer, Askin's sarcoma, was diagnosed. This time he was given fourteen days to live.

The chances of me surviving both these illnesses is the equivalent of winning the lottery four times in a row with the same numbers.

But he miraculously survived and this terrible bump in the road led to some amazing life insights that set him on an unanticipated adventure.

After spending some of his early college and young adult years chasing a range of possibilities from molecular biology and immunology to psychology, he realized he needed to take the time to look deep within to understand his relationship with cancer. School was not his path. He dropped out of a doctoral program to pursue a route that allowed him to use his mind and body together to do something that no one has ever done before: He decided to become the first cancer survivor to climb Everest. On one functional lung.

Sean went on to climb the highest peaks in Africa, Europe, South America, Australia, Antarctica, and North America, known as the Seven Summits. And he didn't stop there. Sean competed in Hawaii's Iron Man Competition and went to the South Pole and the North Pole. On his North Pole expedition, he brought a film crew that captured his quest.

This is his story.

Sean Swarner: The Conversation

This conversation has been edited, but there's so much more to the story! When you have time, scan the QR code and you can listen to the original unedited conversation and view videos and photos of each guest. Or just visit BumpInTheRoad.us/Readers-Portal/ and sign in.

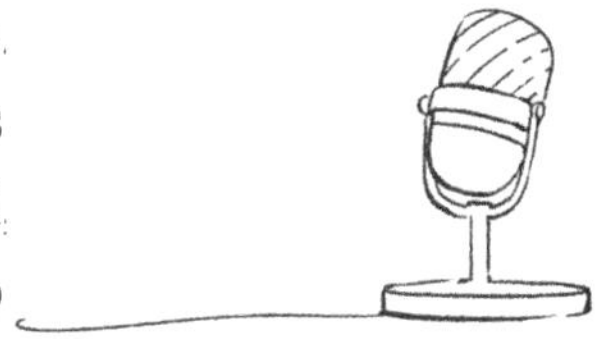

Sean: I was born in a small town in Ohio. I was your typical Midwest guy. There was a bean field or a soy field in my backyard, depending on the season. And I was into everything. I was into every sport. I was into every bit of trouble that you can think of. And as I grew older, I realized that if I was smart enough, I could still do those things I wanted to do, but not get caught!

I became smarter as I grew older until I was thirteen. I was in the eighth grade, and that's when my entire life changed. I suffered an injury to my left knee. When I came down from a layup in basketball, it snapped. That injury triggered every other joint in my body to go haywire.

A few days later, I looked like the Pillsbury Dough Boy, and mom and dad had no idea what was going on. They took me from Willard to Columbus, Ohio. And when I was down there, I had a bone marrow test and a CT scan.

And that's when they found out that I had advanced stage four Hodgkin's lymphoma. I realized at thirteen that my life was going to be completely different.

When my friends were worried about chasing girls and collecting baseball cards, I was worried about waking up the next morning. I started looking at things differently, from a different perspective.

Pat: That's a huge paradigm shift to have at such a young age.

Sean: Especially because at that age, hormones are kicking in. My friends were growing hair in unusual places on their bodies. I was losing my hair and was sixty pounds overweight from the chemo.

I remember one afternoon, I took a shower and all of my hair fell out at the same time. I collapsed to my hands and knees. I was crying my eyeballs out, pulling chunks of hair out of the drain so that the water could go down.

I decided I didn't want to die. I wanted to live.

But in that same moment, I was thinking of what my friends were doing, getting ready for school.

And that was the paradigm shift. What my friends were worried about didn't mean anything to me.

Pat: Did this paradigm shift come to you quickly? Or was it something that took a little while to settle into your perspective?

Sean: To be honest with you, it's still settling in. That was when I was thirteen. I'm forty-five now.

It's going to be a life-long lesson, I think. But the paradigm shift happened at that moment on the bottom of the shower floor. I realized I could either fight for my life or give up and die. Obviously, the latter wasn't an option. So, I chose to live.

Pat: I think a lot of people hit a point in life and face that conscious choice to live or give up. It's not about 'not dying.' It is about living and everything that that means, with all the passion that goes with it.

Sean: Absolutely. Every year I take a group up to Kilimanjaro as a fundraiser for a cancer charity. And so many people always look at it from the wrong perspective. They think 'I'm going to conquer that mountain.'

You're not going to conquer that mountain; you're going to conquer yourself.

I think a lot of people need to do the hard work of looking at themselves in the mirror and figuring out who they are, what they want to be, and at the core, what their values are.

We often stray off the path because we don't have those values in line.

And when you're going down your path in life and suddenly you start to feel a little dissonant, you feel a little off, you feel anxious, you feel anxiety, you feel fear. I honestly think it's because you're not following who you are; you're following other people. And as soon as you start going after other people's goals and you start following what other people want you to do, you lose who you are.

Pat: I totally agree with you. You went through cancer twice, as a child, didn't you?

Sean: I did. I was in remission for a year from the first one, and I was going in for a checkup when they found a completely unrelated primary tumor. It was osteosarcoma and I was sixteen.

With the first cancer, they told my parents I had three months to live. The second time around, they told my parents that I had fourteen days.

I remember just lying in the hospital. A clergyman came in and started giving me my last rites. It kind of reminded me of the Monty Python movie where they're saying, "Bring out your dead, bring out your dead."

They put a guy on the truck. He looks at him and says, "I'm not dead yet."

And they reply, "But you will be soon."

As far as any research shows, I'm the only person in the world who've ever had both Hodgkin's and Askin's sarcoma (osteosarcoma). The chances of me surviving both those illnesses is the equivalent to winning the lottery four times in a row with the same numbers.

Pat: So how do you go from surviving such brutal treatment to climbing Everest with one lung? That's beyond a story.

Sean: After I graduated from high school, in that small town I was known as "cancer boy." Everybody knew my story. I think there were 112 people in my senior class.

I went to college and put it all behind me. I didn't want to be known as cancer boy. I buried the whole experience and I turned into Belushi from Animal House. I had a wonderful time and I jokingly told my parents, "Thank you for the $100,000 four-and-a-half-year-long party that I had."

I started off studying molecular biology and immunology, but it's incredibly difficult to get a decent grade when you don't study. So, I switched to psychology. I took the GRE, and I moved to Jacksonville, Florida, to get my master's and my doctorate in counseling psych. I wanted to be a psycho-oncologist, but I didn't do any research on what cancer meant to *me*. I just didn't do it. It takes a strong person to look deep within themselves to understand their relationship with cancer.

I dropped out of school. I just needed some time off and I realized that school just wasn't my path. Then I did some research and realized that I wanted to use my mind and my body together to do something that no human had ever done before. My brother and I found that no cancer survivor had ever climbed Everest.

I figured if I was going to be the first person to do that, why not do it for the right reasons?

I wanted to use Everest as the highest platform in the world to scream hope and to give back to the cancer community.

Pat: How did you train for Everest?

Sean: Well, good question. I moved to Colorado, where I live now, and I literally did something every single day because:

Consistency is more important than intensity.

A lot of people train their bodies.

They train their muscles to get bigger and stronger,
but the most important muscle is rarely trained.
And that's the six-inch gap between your ears.

What I did every night was I visualized myself on this summit and I used as many senses as possible because that taps into your emotions. And your emotions are closely linked to your subconscious.

In my mind, before I even left Colorado to go over to Nepal, I was already successful. I had that emotional attachment to the end result. So, when I was on the mountain, it was almost like déjà vu.

Pat: That's really interesting. I've also had some experiences with visualizations, and I agree, you must use all your senses. They can be incredibly powerful. It's something that I'm really surprised we don't teach in terms of life skills.

Sean: I think it's because it has the stigma that people think if I sit in a corner and I wish for something hard enough, and I see it hard enough, it's going to happen. You have to put in the hard work. It's not just going to happen by magic. I think so many people just don't understand; there's that disconnect.

Many people are closed-minded. They like to control everything. And you can't control a mountain. Look at Kilimanjaro. Some people go there and say, "I'm going to conquer that mountain."

If it's you against Mother Nature, she's
going to kick your butt every single time.

Pat: After years of soaring, I have learned enormous respect for Mother Nature. What are some of the common things that people run into on a climb like Kilimanjaro?

Sean: I would say two of the biggest things would be they mentally defeat themselves, and they don't have that self-confidence. They let the voices of other people control what they think is possible for them as to what they think is possible for themselves.

Pat: Wow. That goes to life in general, doesn't it?

Sean: Absolutely.

The mountains are a great reflection, a great analogy for life.

Pat: For our listeners who may not know, you have climbed the Seven Summits, the highest mountain peak on each continent. What common challenges did you see with each of those climbs?

Sean: The common challenge is psychological and logistical. In the case of Antarctica, just getting there is a pain in the rear end, because you have to wait for perfect weather. There are no airports. You land on a blue ice runway that takes forever. The pilot can't step on the brakes because he has to use the engines to slow down. If you step on the brakes you're going to start sliding. So, getting there is odd. Then there is the cold, and you're battling the elements in yourself the whole time.

Pat: The North Pole, that was another trip you did recently. One of the things that always stuck with me about that trip was the fact that the North Pole is an ice floe. And it moves. So, you could move ahead twenty miles one day, but if the flow moved backward twenty miles that day, you're still in the same spot.

Sean: Exactly. If you can just picture the world as a giant glass of ice water, the ice floats on the top and that's essentially the northern polar ice cap. Let's say you swirl your glass in a circle. The ice goes with it, and then you stop, that motion of the water underneath still moves the ice. It's the samc thing on a much, much larger scale where the ice cap is floating. And there are millions, if not billions, of ice chunks floating around, running into each other.

If you plan it right, you can go with the current. So, you could ski ten miles and then float two miles more while you're sleeping. You just covered two miles in your dreams!

Pat: You did a film on that trip, didn't you?

Sean: We did. It's on Amazon Prime now, it's called *True North, The Sean Swarner Story*. And it was filmed by a company called The Workshop based out of Philadelphia. The footage they captured is breathtaking. Somehow, they managed to make eighty degrees below zero look tolerable.

Pat: What did you learn from that film experience?

Sean: I learned that when it gets to eighty below zero, camera lens oil freezes!

Johnny Walker sent me a bottle of Johnny Walker blue label, and it said, "Sean Swarner Best Served On Ice." I had it in my sled because on expeditions like that, it's traditional to celebrate with some whiskey.

The night before we were going to make it to the North Pole, I think we were five miles away. We knew we were going to make it the next day. I pulled out the bottle and looked at it just to get excited, and believe it or not, it was so cold outside that the bottle was frozen solid. I stuck the square bottle into an old sock and surrounded it with some extra hand warmers. I had to warm up the whiskey to drink it!

Pat: Slight change of topic. I was looking at your blog this morning. And one of the things that you said is:

Understand your intrinsic motivators.

And I think that has so much wisdom in it. Would you talk a little bit about that?

Sean: One of the things that people don't realize is that if you're going after something that someone else wants for you, you're losing *yourself.*

Intrinsic motivators go back to what I call personal core values. And if you can tap into your personal core values, you have more purpose.

You have that personal motivation,
and you can perpetually motivate yourself.

If people just understand what their intrinsic motivators are,
they can be your guiding principles in life.

Thoughts For You to Ponder

Can you name three of your intrinsic motivators?

What do you say to yourself that is self-defeating?

What's your greatest mountain?

Key Takeaways

- Your reaction to events is a choice
- Align yourself with your innermost values
- You're not going to conquer that mountain; you're going to conquer yourself

CHAPTER THIRTEEN

Putting Your Best Foot Forward

"I think it's like a second chance that I just want to grab hold of."

–SARAH DRANSFIELD

Learning to walk. The need for balance and rhythm. The strength it requires to go the distance. Step by step.

Learning to walk is both an action and a metaphor. It's about taking life one step at a time. It's about daring to move forward in small increments. It's about moving into uncertainty.

Uncertainty is the companion of an engaged life. It recognizes that each moment, each step, offers an act of creation. Or re-creation. It's not often we get a second chance.

With a second chance at life, what would you do?

Reflections on My Life Circa 2022

When I was younger, I wanted certainty. I followed a linear path that suggested companionship and security. I lived for a future that never happened. I worked, I achieved, I married. My careful plans all turned out to be an illusion. And in the maelstrom that followed, I was forced to shred my elusive and imaginary future and tread an unseen path to an unseen destination.

Had I not taken a chance on that ride in Calistoga; had I not stormed off from Kampel to an unknown airfield in an angry rush; had I not taken Whiskey Oscar on that cross-country trip, I would not be where I am today.

There is an even longer litany of what ifs in my path, accompanied by many bumps ranging from business betrayal to cancer. But in those bumps, I reconnected with my creativity and I was able to resurrect my passion for writing. I stumbled upon a new interest, photography, that would eventually lead me to Africa. From a series of travels and events came the podcast, and now this book. In uncertainty, step by step, I found possibility.

I have taken risks and chances that some would say are unwise. But in those steps into the unknown, I found a life experience that, on occasion, touches the transcendental. It is in this magic that I strive to live, and I would not trade that path for the mere illusion of certainty.

There is a part of me that likes routine, just like anyone else. I'm fairly disciplined. I rise at 4:45 in the morning, read something inspirational, find five new things to be grateful for, meditate, make a matcha latte, and start the day. I like my routine. I don't really want to change it.

But sometimes, change is thrust upon us and the comfort of our routines crumble. But we rebuild. We find a different path; one which we might never have imagined. It happened to me. And it happened to Sarah Dransfield.

Meet My Guest Sarah Dransfield: Model, Volunteer, Adventurer

At just sixteen years old, Sarah Dransfield was diagnosed with osteosarcoma. After nearly a year of hospitalized treatment, the outlook was still grim. Chemo wasn't working. An amputation of her right leg was needed to stem the spread of the cancer.

Where does a teenager go with a life interrupted not just by cancer, but by losing a leg?

Sarah's story is one of courage, perseverance, and evolution. The young girl that started out as shy and quiet now does interviews and lives a rich life. She has met the Queen and modeled for *Vogue Italia*. She's sky dived and rides a bike.

All with a prosthetic leg.

In addition to modeling, Sarah volunteers at the Laura Crane Youth Cancer Trust, which helps teens throughout the UK and Ireland. Her life has changed a lot in the last ten years, but the loneliness and isolation of cancer hasn't. She gives back to help those coming after her; to help them find their own path through such a life-disrupting experience.

From dating to working, Sarah has found her path. And she's found a peer group of young women who support each other. They are all amputees. They call themselves "Legs, Legs, Legs."

Sarah Dransfield: The Conversation

This conversation has been edited, but there's so much more to the story! When you have time, scan the QR code and you can listen to the original unedited conversation and view videos and photos of each guest. Or just visit BumpInTheRoad.us/Readers-Portal/ and sign in.

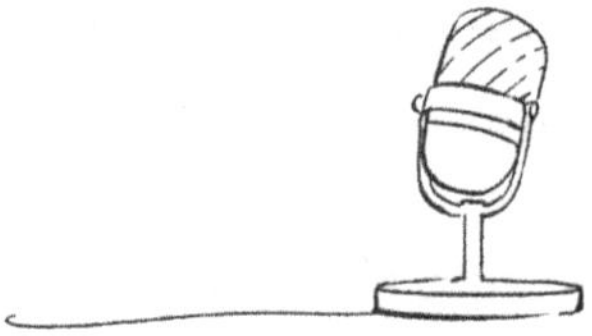

Sarah: I'm Sarah. I'm from Huddersfield in the United Kingdom. My story starts in 2012. I'd been on holiday with my family to Thailand. When I stepped off the plane from Thailand, I felt this strong pain in my knee. I wasn't sure what it was or if I had just sat funny on the plane. But this pain carried on for three months. It just got increasingly worse as time went on.

I was diagnosed with bone cancer in March on my mom's birthday. My parents took me to the doctor, and they explained that I had osteosarcoma, which is a form of bone cancer, which generally happens in young men.

Pat: And you were just sixteen at this point, right?

Sarah: Yeah, just sixteen. So, it was a massive shock because I thought I'd just sprained my leg or somehow injured it. I never thought it would be cancer.

Pat: What went through your mind? I can't even imagine.

Sarah: Literally, first thing I said was, "Am I going to die?'

The doctor who diagnosed me said I'd lose a year out of my life. Potentially, they might be able to scrape the cancer off my knee and I'd be fine, or I might lose my legs. So, all in that conversation, I had everything going on.

I had chemotherapy for a full year. It was a really intense year. I was so sick with the chemo. The doctor said that I was the worst case they'd ever seen. Every anti-sickness drug they gave me, nothing worked. I lost a lot of weight, and I had a feeding tube to feed me. But that didn't do much, because obviously you're quite sick when you have chemotherapy, and then that kept coming up and it was just like a vicious cycle.

Pat: In the midst of all that, what are you thinking?

Sarah: Oh, I don't know. It's all a bit of a whirlwind now. I think at the time I was just going along with it, thinking I must do this, I have to have this treatment, even if it's making me so ill. But I was just thinking I hope it's making me better at the same time.

Pat: But the chemo didn't work, did it?

Sarah: No. I was supposed to have the bone in my knee replaced with metal so I could save my leg. But the tumor was deep into my bone and near the nerve. And there's a big artery that runs down your leg. It was very close to that. If they did operate, it would be really risky.

So, the best chance for survival was to have an amputation above my knee.

That's what I had to go with. But I just thought, no, I can't have an amputation. There's no chance. I don't know how I'd live without my leg.

Pat: I don't think you come to terms with something like that in a week or a month or even in years.

Sarah: No, not at all. It takes a long time. I think for me, even when I did have the amputation, for many weeks and months after I was still having chemotherapy. So, I was still in the midst of everything, just getting on with it. But I think when you're back to just being on your own, I think that's when it hits you the most.

Pat: Was it hard adjusting to a new leg?

Sarah: It was really hard. First of all, I didn't get a leg straight away. My leg was quite swollen. It had to reduce in size before

I could try one out. So, I was going to physio whilst having my chemotherapy, which was tough. The thought of having to learn to walk whilst going through the treatment still was quite a lot to deal with. I did what I could. After my chemotherapy finished, I focused on learning to walk again. And it took me quite a long time to get to where I am now.

Pat: What's the hardest part? Is it getting the prosthetic fitted properly? Is it balance? Is it mobility? What are the things that you have to think about?

Sarah: I think it's everything, really. Balance is a big one because you're so used to being able to stand on your two legs.

I'm brilliant at balancing now.

I think that's just come over time. But the balance when you're learning to work with your prosthetic, it is different because it's a foreign object. It's not your leg, is it? So that was hard.

Walking with a prosthetic takes twice as much energy as a normal person walking. And building up my muscle to be able to wear the prosthetic was a long journey, because my leg was shrinking down every six months to a year. I'd have to get a new socket for the prosthetic quite often, which meant trips back and forth to the hospital quite a lot. But I've got to the point where it's stabilized a lot now, which is a good thing.

Pat: When all this started, what were your plans? Were you going to college? What were you thinking about doing?

Sarah: I had just started college in September and in March I was diagnosed. I was studying psychology and applied science. I wasn't really sure where I was going, but I knew I liked caring for people.

When I finished treatment the following March, I went back to the college in September.

It was so hard because all my friends had left.

I found it really difficult. I was quite on my own. I was now in my brother's year, who was two years younger than me. But I felt so much older with what I'd just been through and everything I'd just dealt with. That was a difficult time.

I was also still learning to walk at that point, and I had crutches and people just didn't know me. I looked like a different person. I had short hair, I put weight on, I was just not who I was before. I didn't really have any friends there.

Pat: The social isolation with cancer is something everybody talks about. I can't imagine how hard it had to be. Did you have any sort of peer group anywhere?

Sarah: Going through my treatment, I'd made friends in the hospital. We've got a charity over here called the Teenage Cancer Trust and they have wards in the hospital for teenagers. So, I was able to make friends with people I could relate to.

But with my friends from school, it was difficult because they were still so young themselves. For them to deal with me having cancer and understanding what I was going through, they just couldn't.

Pat: This is a really hard question to ask because I need to be more specific, but I can't be. How has cancer changed your outlook? And I know there are so many pieces to this.

Sarah: It's a massive question. I think it's changed my outlook massively. I always think back and wonder how my life would've been if I didn't have cancer. Would I be living a parallel life to what I'm living now? I don't know what I'd be doing.

It has changed me. I want to try and make the most of life now and do everything that I can. I want to travel more. I could have died back in 2012.

I think it's like a second chance that I just want to grab hold of.

I appreciate my family and my friends more. Any time that I spend with them is precious. The experience changed me massively, but

it's changed me for the better.

I was quite shy before. Now I do talks and things like that. I would never have dreamt of doing that before. I now look different. Coming to terms with that, and speaking about my story, is something I would never have done. So yeah, it's massively changed my outlook.

Pat: I understand you have a spread in *Italian Vogue.*

Sarah: I do! I'm quite shocked about that.

Pat: Tell us about that. That's really cool.

Sarah: It's amazing. I did a photo shoot in a town close to where I live. The shoot was a bit quirky and a bit different. They sent the picture out there and

Italian Vogue *picked it up.*

Then the next thing I get an email saying, "here's the picture of you in *Italian Vogue.*"

So, quite amazing. Really quite a highlight.

Pat: How did you get into modeling?

Sarah: I'd been looking on Instagram and I'd found a management company that focused on diversity and people with disabilities. I thought, oh, I'll apply and I'll see what happens. I wasn't sure whether they'd want me or not. But they did.

My first job for them was for River Island clothing. I was suddenly down in London doing a photo shoot.

I was just going along with it and hoping for the best. But then I went down to London for another job.

I went into the River Island store on Oxford Street, and I saw myself behind the counter on this big billboard.

I was so shocked, but I did feel quite proud.

Pat: Have you gotten a lot of feedback from people in the disability community about your modeling?

Sarah: I've got Instagram and I post when I do something new. I've got quite a lot of followers who are disabled, and they love seeing it. They think:

It's great that disability is being shown out there and being made to be normal, which it should be.

Pat: What do you do about dating and things like that?

Sarah: When I was first told about my amputation, I thought, "Oh my God, no one is going to love me. I'm never going to get a boyfriend, and why would they want me with one leg?"

For a long time, I just thought it wasn't possible.

I started to go out with my friends on the weekends and get dressed up. And I think by the time I got to twenty, I'd been on a few dates. But when I was twenty-one, my mom saw that you could apply for the show *First Date*.

It's quite a big show over here. You basically have a date, and you don't know who you're going to be meeting. There's a team that works behind the scenes. They work hard to match you with someone that they think you'd be compatible with.

So, they got to know me. And then they got to know the person I'd be going on a date with. The date was in London, and it was filmed. And that's where I met my boyfriend, Phil, who I have now been with for nearly four years. That was quite an incredible journey.

Pat: If you could rewrite your story, would you?

Sarah: Oh, that's a tricky one. I don't think I would because I just think of things that I've done since.

I've done so much; I've had so many opportunities.

And yeah, I deal with my disability on a daily basis. There's no hiding away from it. But I think all the things I've done have just made me who I am now.

I feel like maybe I was meant to be who I am now.

A few years ago, I was lucky enough to meet the Queen. I would never have met the Queen otherwise. I've done all sorts of things, like sailing with a cancer charity. I'm an ambassador for another cancer charity. I've done skydives and things that I would never have thought to do.

Pat: You went skydiving?

Sarah: Yeah, I was with an instructor. And obviously I couldn't wear my prosthetic because it's a bit dangerous, like falling from the sky with my prosthetic on.

Pat: It's a little dangerous falling from the sky without one, too.

Sarah: Yeah. Never mind with one on! That was quite difficult in itself because I had to use my crutches to get up onto the plane. And then when we landed it was how do I get about without my leg? So, it was a bit more than just your average sky dive.

Pat: If you were to give some advice to somebody facing a bump in the road in general, what advice would you give to them?

Sarah: I think I would say,

Try and talk to the people that you love.

I always found that talking to my family helped me the most. Having something to focus on or something to look forward to also helped. If you know in a few weeks' time you've got like a little something to look forward to, seeing a friend, going somewhere, going for a walk, anything, I think that really can help you get through a tough patch.

Try and stay as positive as you can.

Finding people that are in a similar position really helped and it is still helping me now. I've got a group of friends and we call ourselves Legs, Legs, Legs. We've all got one leg. We're a group of young ladies, and if we ever need anyone to talk to, we've always got each other.

Thoughts For You to Ponder

What's your greatest disability?

How has it challenged and changed you?

What bump have you hit that led to new experiences? In retrospect, would you avoid that bump if you could?

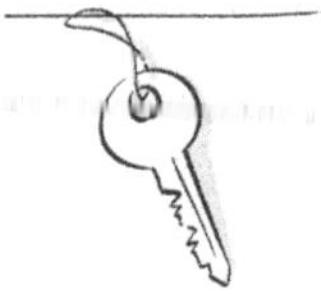

Key Takeaways

- Disability is not abnormal; it's all around us, in all sorts of ways
- Challenges are an opportunity for a more conscious and meaningful life
- Uncertainty is possibility

CHAPTER FOURTEEN

From Hope to Trust

"I absolutely bought into the concept that you had to choose between science and spirituality because the two could not coexist."

–MARY NEAL, MD.

In the next two chapters, I have omitted my reflections on life because I honestly don't think I can add anything meaningful to these stories. While I've had life-changing bumps that sent me on a quest for peace and spiritual meaning, I stand in awe of these next two guests.

In each of these stories, an event comes along that rocks my guests' perception of their universe. For both Mary Neal, M.D. and David Maginley, it was a near death experience.

For Mary Neal, the experience creating an opening, a knowing, that challenged her preconceived notions of the world and challenged her to be open to a greater universe.

Here is her story.

Meet My Guest, Mary Neal, M.D.: Spine Surgeon, Kayaker, Parent

What happens when a pragmatic and analytical scientist experiences something beyond her scientific paradigm?

Mary Neal, M.D. is an accomplished orthopedic spine surgeon. She went to UCLA Medical School, did a residency at USC, and later became the director of spine surgery at USC.

In 1999, Mary was kayaking in Chile with her husband and friends. As an experienced kayaker, the rapids and ten-to-fifteen-foot waterfalls on the Fuy River were well within her ability. But when one kayaker blocked the obvious route over a waterfall, Mary was forced to detour and take another, more dangerous path. At the base of the waterfall, she and her kayak were pulled underwater and pinned under a powerful cascade of eight to ten feet of water.

She couldn't move under the force of the river, which bent her body in half and both legs backwards from the knee. Underwater for thirty minutes, Mary Neal, M.D., orthopedic spine surgeon and mother of four, drowned and had a spiritual experience that would change her life.

The sequence of events that led to her rescue were improbable, at best.

CPR restarted her heart. Several young Chilean men appeared out of the jungle and took her to a nearby road. Her husband, who had passed on the day's kayaking, miraculously connected with Mary as she was being loaded into an ambulance, in a place where ambulances didn't exist. The details of her incredible journey are in her book, *To Heaven and Back.*

Mary finally made it back to Jackson Hole, where her internist doubted she would survive the night. In addition to the orthopedic injuries, she had advanced pneumonia and acute respiratory distress syndrome, a reactive swelling of the lung tissue which interferes with the ability to exchange oxygen.

Mary survived, but she faced months of healing and rehab, during which she tried to make sense of the experience.

As a surgeon and analytical thinker, she said:

> *"I tried to come up with a medical scientific*
> *explanation for what I'd experienced. . .*
> *I was trying to disprove my own experiences."*

But her only conclusion could be that she had been sent back to her body from a place she called Heaven.

Mary Neal, M.D.: The Conversation

This conversation has been edited, but there's so much more to the story! When you have time, scan the QR code and you can listen to the original unedited conversation and view videos and photos of each guest. Or just visit BumpInTheRoad.us/Readers-Portal/ and sign in.

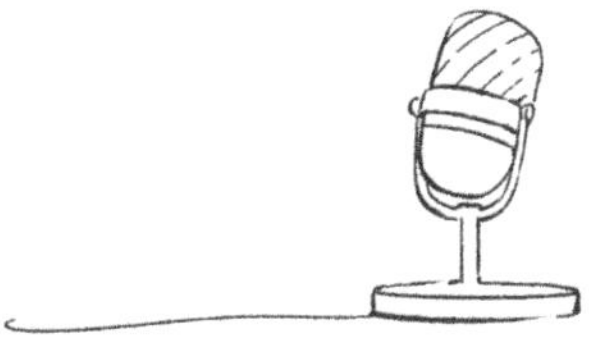

Mary: I am an orthopedic spine surgeon. I would say I was a nominal Christian before I had the experience I'm about to describe. And when I say that, I mean that I was raised in the American Midwest, and like most Midwestern young people I was taken to church on Sunday morning and then Monday morning I went back to my life. And there was never a sense of integration or gee, how can this actually help you lead a joyful life? It just wasn't that kind of a thing. It was basically a routine. And when I went off to college and medical school,

> *I absolutely bought into the concept that*
> *you had to choose between science and*
> *spirituality because the two could not coexist.*

And I am a scientist. I've always been a scientist. I have a very analytical, somewhat skeptical, a little bit cynical brain. I was fully committed to science and intellect over any sense of faith or spirituality.

I finished medical school. I went through my surgical training, and I became a spine surgeon, and I ran the spine service at the University of Southern California. I was married and had four young children.

My husband and I went to Chile in South America to go kayaking. Kayaking is something that we have done for many, many years.

On what was going to be our last day, we decided to paddle on a section of river that's well known for its waterfalls. And although I'm going to call them waterfalls, it's not Niagara Falls. There are drops of ten to fifteen feet, which for an experienced kayaker is fun and challenging and exhilarating, but it's not crazy. It was certainly within our skillset.

My husband that morning, for the first and only time in his life, had an experience of horrible back pain, so he did not go with us that day, but he dropped us off and we started down the river.

The first couple of drops were fine. Then we came to the first more significant drop. Because it was early, we decided to go over a smaller part of the waterfall. This river, unlike many of the rivers in the U.S., was very high flow. And the topography was such that there weren't eddies or areas of slow water where you could sort of pull out and regroup or change your plan.

I started down the river. There was another American client who sort of bobbled past me, and her boat ended up sideways in the drop that we were going to go over. My only option was to veer away, and in veering away I was swept over the main part of the waterfall. As I looked at the bottom, I could tell that it was not going to be fun. What I thought would happen is that I would hit the bottom, be flipped upside down, and probably not be able to right myself because of the turbulence and the hydraulics.

I assumed that I would push myself out of my kayak and tumble around for a couple of minutes before being spit out downstream. But instead

what happened was nothing I could
ever in my wildest imagination come up with.

My boat went down and became pinned underwater. The boat and I were then immediately buried under eight to ten feet of water.

I am a spine surgeon. I'm not sure that I relish high-stress situations, but I'm very comfortable with them. So, I didn't panic or anything like that. In addition, I am an absolute water person. A good day for me is doing anything in or on the water. But I will also say that I had a lifetime fear of drowning. I thought that drowning would be the most horrible way to die ever. And there I was, drowning. The irony of it was not lost on me.

I am very pragmatic. I knew my predicament. I knew the likelihood of rescue was very slim and I thought about my options. And at that point, the only thing that came over me was really a very sincere request, desire, prayer that God's will be done.

I know that that sounds like a very passive thing. Like, oh, well, you're going to die, so give your life over to God. But it wasn't that. I don't know how to verbally express the difference, but it was a very active choice that yes, God, your will be done. And I am totally on board with whatever that outcome is.

The minute I asked that, I was immediately overcome with a very physical sensation of being held and comforted and reassured by Christ that everything would be fine. And I was so shocked. I was no Christian zealot. I'm pretty skeptical. But I was so overcome with love. It was nothing I could ever express in our vocabulary.

I certainly never thought about what would happen after death. I think, based on my childhood upbringing, I hoped there was something more, whatever that means. But I'd never thought about it specifically.

If someone had asked me about the life review, I would've come up with a Hollywood version, where your life flashes across the sky and you feel great about some things and not so great about others, and maybe have a little empathy. But this life review had nothing to do with any of the destructive emotions, guilt, remorse, regret, or anything like that. It had everything to do with understanding and grace. And grace is the only word I can really use because it's everything to do with love.

I understood everything about my past story, my life story. I had this absolute understanding of how that particular event came to be.

And what I discovered is that it was not a matter of forgiving.

What I discovered is that when you understand,
there is no destructive emotion.

It was absolutely life-changing for me because it gave me a very different understanding of people and human interactions. And that old saying, hurtful words or actions come from a place of pain, it's true.

I was still my pragmatic questioning self. I took a minute and said this must be some bizarre hallucination. Was I in an air pocket? Was I breathing? Was I still conscious? Was I unconscious? I ran through this whole self-assessment exam. I thought about my breathing. I was really not breathing. I mean, it's water.

At a certain point, I felt like I was a manta ray, beautifully intertwined with the water. It was a wonderful feeling. I came to the conclusion that I was not just conscious, I was more conscious. I was not alive; I was more alive.

There was this incredible shift in time. There was no sense of the past or the present. It was entirely all about the moment.

The current was pulling my body over the front deck of the boat, and I could feel my knees bend backwards and bones break. Eventually, my spirit broke free from my body. I rose up and out of the river and was greeted by a group of people, spirits, beings. Those names mean different things to different people, so I never really know what to call them. There's no way to describe them with our vocabulary either because:

They were wearing these pearlescent robes
that were woven together with fibers of love.

They started to take me down this pathway toward this incredible domed structure. I don't know how to describe it. This pathway existed in the middle of nothingness, and it was woven together with every color of the universe and colors that I'd never seen. It was a simultaneous purity of color, purity of these thousands of thousands of flowers and the aroma of flowers.

It all sounds pretty crazy, but it was something that spoke to me, and I absolutely believe that God speaks to each of us in the way that we will understand and presents to each of us at the time of our death the experience that we will understand, that will make us feel loved and make us feel like we're home.

And that was my overwhelming experience
and feeling, which is that I was home.

I was in my real home, my true home. It was like I'd been on this incredible adventure to Earth, and now I was home.

We eventually got to the end of this pathway and we were at this archway for what seemed like many, many hours. While I was there, I had the sense that I understood everything. I understood quantum physics, which I don't understand. All I had to do was think about something and I could understand it.

I understood not the divine nature of God, but I definitely understood the divine order of our universe, how we are all interconnected, how every action makes a difference, every human interaction, every interaction with everything. Plants, animals, people, everything we do and say matters.

I kind of knew that was a point of no return. I kept trying to go over the threshold and was told it wasn't my time. I had more work to do on Earth and I had to go back to my body.

I objected. I had been initially reassured by Christ that everything was going to be fine. My husband would be fine. My kids would be fine regardless of whether I lived or died. It's hard for me to acknowledge that I didn't actually want to come back, because I had a great life. I had every reason in the world to desperately want to come back. But when juxtaposed to the purity and intensity of God's love and the love of our home,

I said, no, my journey's over. I'm here to stay.
But I was kicked out.

I was taken back down the pathway, and I was given a laundry list of expectations and things that I had to do.

It's a long story from there to coming back to Wyoming for medical care. It's a story filled with miracles.

I underwent several surgeries and many months of rehab. And during those many months, I started the process of trying to figure out what that experience was all about. There were things that happened that really are inexplicable. I spent months going over all my medical records, talking to the people who had been at the river and in the emergency room, and going back and looking at the literature. I somewhat desperately tried to come up with any medical or scientific explanation for what I had experienced.

I was trying to disprove my own experiences because I knew that if I could, then I could ignore everything I'd been told about things I still had to do. None of which I wanted to do.

And I would be able to ignore what I'd been told about my son's coming death.

In the end, I was forced to concede that all my experiences had been true and real spiritual experiences.

And one of the things that it did for me ultimately is make me realize that:

This idea that science and spirituality are binary is false.

Pat: How do you learn to live with an experience like this? And how does it change you?

Mary: It changes every part of a person. It can't do anything short of that because it transforms your hope.

That one truth changes everything about our experience on Earth. It changes everything about birth, life, death. It can't help but change everything because if there really is life after death, you have to start asking what does that mean for my life? What am I doing here? What's the purpose? It changes everything about your human interactions and everything about your understanding and reaction to life and to life events.

I know that for me, it transformed any hope or faith I had that God is real and present, and God has made some promises to us. There is absolute trust in those promises. And with that absolute trust, I have discovered a life that is joy-filled and I believe we are meant to live lives of joy.

I don't have regret. I don't have guilt. I don't have anger. I don't have bitterness. And of course,

So many people live in the past and their past defines their present and it limits their future.

I don't have that, because I know that if I could understand the backstory of myself and anyone else involved in the past, I would feel nothing but empathy for myself, empathy for other people. I would feel nothing but love.

It's an absolute grace and a complete reconciliation with people who you've hurt and people who hurt you. Those negative destructive emotions don't exist. That leaves me with the present and in the present. I still make plans, but I hold all those plans very loosely because I know that if my plans don't work out, it's because God has a different, probably better plan.

And so, I'm able to exist in the moment. And I believe that's where joy is found; in each moment.

Pat: Does it take courage to live a fearless life?

Mary: I believe it takes trust. And I think every person is able to make that transition. It doesn't require a profound spiritual experience. It requires an open heart and an open mind. And the ability to question whether things in your life could be spiritual in nature.

I believe that fear, which is the root of so many problems, does not exist in the presence of God's love.

I don't think it requires courage to step out fearlessly. I think it requires trust.

Thoughts For You to Ponder

How would changing your world view from "hope" to "trust" change your life?

How has coincidence or synchronicity come into your life? Did you listen?

Have you ever been guilty of living in the past? How has it limited your future?

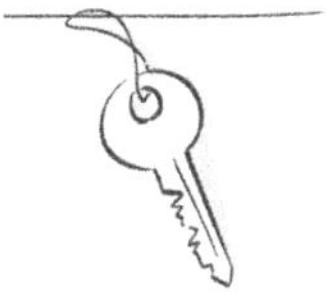

Key Takeaways

- The world is far greater than we can imagine
- A linear train of thought dependent upon absolute proof may limit your perspective
- Trust in a greater spiritual presence will change your world

CHAPTER FIFTEEN

What If We See Only 0.004% of the Universe?

"How can you become love?"

–DAVID MAGINLEY

David's story resonates on so many levels. From a lifetime of dealing with a rare and deadly cancer to the knowledge and faith in his calling as an interfaith minister, David's wisdom and humility are extraordinary. So is his perspective of the world. Here is his story.

Meet My Guest, David Maginley: Interfaith Spiritual Pastor

Rev. David Maginley is an interfaith spiritual counselor at the QEII Health Sciences Centre in Halifax, Nova Scotia, and award-winning author of *Beyond Surviving: Cancer and Your Spiritual Journey*. He is featured in the documentaries *Here Right Now* and *When You Die*. David has also survived cancer four times, which resulted in a profound near-death experience and explorations in the connection of body, mind, and spirit.

His book *Beyond Surviving* is a beautiful, eloquent exploration of his experiences as a reverend, as a patient, and as a human looking for greater meaning in life. His near death experience challenged and expanded his reality, and this discussion may ask the same of you.

Join us as we discuss his experiences, insights, and revelations regarding life, death, and life afterwards.

David Maginley: The Conversation

This conversation has been edited, but there's so much more to the story! When you have time, scan the QR code and you can listen to the original unedited conversation and view videos and photos of each guest. Or just visit BumpInTheRoad.us/Readers-Portal/ and sign in.

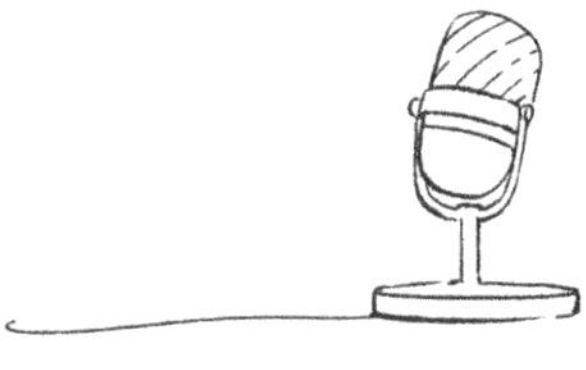

David: It's been an interesting road for me. I'm a chaplain for cancer patients in palliative intensive care. I work with death and dying and suffering and hope and mortality five days a week. But I seem to be oddly comfortable in that.

I think that's due in large part to the fact that I've had cancer four times. I was seventeen years old when I was diagnosed with a strange, rare tumor called paraganglioma. And these little creatures make a Molotov cocktail of adrenaline; enough to cause instant death. When your adrenal gland turns on, for whatever reason—stress or even joy or excitement—that causes the tumor to blow. It only takes about a minute to die from this, because it causes a massive heart attack and your blood pressure spikes through the roof.

Now, I have had many minor explosions which often rendered me unconscious, but never took my life, that occurred when I was seventeen, and then twenty-seven, then thirty-five, then thirty-eight years old. Thankfully, I'm fifty-six years old now, so I think I'm out of the woods, but

cancer taught me how to be awake to the gift of life and work wisely with suffering.

It's an honor to support others as they face those health crises.

It's been quite a journey. I'm grateful for it because I think I've been learning how to not only go through cancer but grow through cancer. And I hope that I can help others do the same.

I've been in parish ministry for ten years. When I was a student training in a parish, I was doing a service, so it was public speaking. Nothing is quite as anxiety-provoking as speaking in public. And my body was telling me that the tumor was being activated and I felt the effect of that: the peripheral flush, dizziness, buzzing in the ears, stomach cramps. And I thought like all the other times that it had kicked in that I could get this under control, but down I went. I was unconscious before I hit the floor and transported.

During this episode, I had a near death experience. This is a surprisingly common phenomenon; one in ten people who have a brush with death will have a mystical experience, like seeing themselves out of their own body or seeing a different realm.

So, I found myself suddenly on a grassy hill and the light was pouring from everything. I could feel every blade of grass as it moved. And I felt one with love, which infused the light. I felt suddenly whole and complete. There wasn't any aspect of myself that I was suppressing.

I felt finally integrated, authentic, congruent, and more alive than I've ever been here.

I knew I was dead, and that wasn't a problem because I was filled with joy and bliss. This is a common and difficult experience to describe.

It goes to the bone and beyond in reshaping who and what you are in your relationship to reality.

I found myself there with a person who felt like my best friend. I can't physically describe him because that really didn't matter, but he was beauty and compassion and love and joy and power. A lot of people say, "Hey, that sounds like Jesus. You're a Christian Pastor, didn't you think it was Jesus?"

And to be honest, I didn't think it was Jesus. I didn't think they would send the boss to see me.

This entity, which was human and yet was not, walked with me on that grassy hill and we had a chat in which basically he said things were going very well. "We are with you, you have a lot to learn, a lot more work to do. You can't stay here, so you have to go back."

Now, I didn't want to go back. There was a tree at the top of that grassy hill, and I wanted with every fiber of my being to run to that tree because I knew if I got there, I would never come back to Earth. It seemed to be a threshold point. I ached to see what was on the other side of that hill. And yet my feet felt like they were moving through mud. There was something in the power of his presence that prevented me from running up to the tree.

So, we just walked, and I basked in the love and the wholeness that I was experiencing. And I said, "I'm not going back. Why would I go back there?"

Life on Earth is a dimension of being that is fragmented. That is compressed. That is dense. That is limited. That is filled with struggle and suffering, which ultimately are the best avenues of growth and learning.

But I didn't want any more of this. And he imparted to me such gentle compassion and enduring understanding, as you would have with a little child who doesn't want to go to bed on Christmas Eve. He just put his hand on my shoulder and he poured this love into me, and he said, "It's okay. We will be with you. You have a lot more work to do. And we will see you later."

And with that, boom! I was back in my body, and that was horrible. Suddenly the density of flesh and the pull of gravity and the sluggishness of thoughts and the poverty of words swallowed all of that joy and that vitality of being more alive than ever. And I immediately began to grieve. I was now separated from that love that had unfolded before me.

Pat: How do you start to make sense of the reality of that experience and integrate it into this life?

David: You do it awkwardly. Most people, me included, don't know what to do with this type of experience. So, you go through more than cognitive dissonance. You go through existential dissonance. You have been pulled from one reality to another, so expansive, and then compressed back into this reality. What do you do with that?

So, like most people, I buried it. I put it away. I didn't tell anyone. Whenever I thought about it, I would feel this longing and homesickness for it. And yet I had to rationalize it somewhere. I had to integrate it. So, you say to yourself, "oh, it wasn't real, just a dream," or "I don't know what to do with it, so I won't do anything with it," but you cannot shake it. Your soul is aching for what you tasted.

And your whole relationship to life is different now.

You know that you are sustained by something much greater. Most people take about ten years to integrate this. Now, it's much faster if they have a support person or someone to help explain it. And you don't tell others right away because you wonder if they're going to think you're crazy. You would think these things would be talked about much more easily, but a lot of people don't, again because they worry others will think they're crazy.

The Institute of Noetic Science did a fantastic survey and a study on this. They were looking at the varieties or the frequency of exceptional or mystical experiences. And in their survey, they found that over 90 percent of people, including scientists, have had an exceptional mystical experience.

If it's real, if we do indeed continue after our bodies do not, if indeed our reality is emanating and sustained from a deeper level or dimension, we might call spiritual, then these must be universal phenomena. It must be common in the human condition.

In other cultures, people talk openly about it. But in Western culture, we compartmentalize it.

It doesn't fit into that materialist mindset.

Pat: You have some statistics in your book that I find really fascinating. You say that 0.004% of reality is visual.

David: Yes. I love exploring the nature of what is reality, and science has informed me on that much more than my faith has.

Science has discovered that all the visible matter in the universe, all the stuff we can see and feel, represents 0.004% of the universe that's within the visible spectrum of light.

Then there are all the other atoms outside the frequency of the visible spectrum. All the atoms in the universe make up 4 percent of the universe. My goodness, then about 25 percent of the universe is something called dark matter. And astrophysicists have only been able to infer the presence and reality of that by its mathematical effects on the calculations of the movement of galactic clusters. The rest of the universe, over 70 percent, is something called energy.

That means that all our assumptions on what is real are based upon 0.004%.

We are exercising great naiveté and hubris when we say that this is all that there is to reality.

I'm excited by that. It offers an intelligent new paradigm for a spiritual conversation.

Pat: Is this a conversation where spirituality and science start to merge?

David: I think that this is a common ground where the dialogue can go much deeper than it ever has before. And in all healthy, spiritual traditions, the emphasis is upon love. How do you love; how do you treat your fellow human beings? How do you love the world? How do you love yourself?

How can you become love?

Because that's the goal of any healthy spiritual tradition. The religions of the world have not emphasized that enough, but I've discovered that your spirituality is not determined so much by the content of your belief as it is by the quality of your love, for God is love.

Those are synonyms. That flips everything on its head and breaks down the walls. And it can be part of the conversation with science, where we explore the question:

What is the nature of consciousness?

Is God a fundamental primary consciousness from which reality emanates? Let's be open to the mystery and be excited about a new dialogue.

Pat: Now, on a more mundane level, after your near-death experience, you took time, a decade or so, as you tried to integrate that into your life. Did it lead to a paradigm change in the way you see things?

David: Yes. And I'm really embarrassed to say that as monumental and foundational as that paradigm shift was, I still sometimes forget that I am a spiritual being having a physical experience. I forget that all the noise of the world is just that; it is noise. Only love is the most essential, important thing, and how we live that out and exercise it in justice and fairness and equity and compassion.

Above all, there must be compassion.

Even with my near-death experience, I forget all this and get caught up in the noise, and I'm as human and flawed as the next person. But it only takes a moment for me to remember my near-death experience and return to that gratitude and that absolute peace and calm and confidence that it's all going be okay.

Pat: Once you have that knowing within you, it seems to me that as long as you can hang onto it, it permanently changes one's perspective on life.

David: Yes, but there are subtle nuances in that. If I try to hang on to it, it tends to slip away. But if I realize that it has me, it's hanging onto me, and I've always been flowing and emanating from it, then I can relax into it.

Then it lives naturally within me. It's important for me to remember that with all my reading and all my training, and even having written a book about this, I have a human brain and I tend to get in my own way. This is where I find that:

The practice of mindfulness and presence are foundational to realigning myself with love.

Pat: One of the things you ask in your book has to do with the whole experience of cancer, and you asked not "why did it happen to me," but "what can I do with it?"

David: Yes. I like the quote from a doctor in there that says, "Don't waste the crisis."

Cancer is a massive bump in the road. The first step is accepting that it is the reality; your new reality. You can't do that right away. You negotiate with your mortality, even with a very treatable cancer. But then you move to, "What am I going do with this?" Because "why me" can spiral into a sense of helplessness.

Asking "what am I going do with this?" is empowering.

It's using a crisis or suffering as the greatest opportunity for growth to evolve into love. That tends to realign your priorities and reshape the whole texture of life.

Pat: And I think something like cancer really focuses your awareness on the wonder of ordinary and simple things. That alone is a paradigm shift from this so-called reality that we live in, where we're bombarded by snippets of usually negative news. One must stop and realize that it really is an amazing, wonderful world. And wow, what a road trip this is.

David: Yeah. What a wild ride! We would like it to be without the bumps, but if it weren't for the bumps in my life, I would not have grown into the man I am now. And I'm pretty happy with that.

Pat: Well, that brings up an interesting question. You have been through a lot; would you rewrite any part of your story?

David: Oh, what a good question. There are days I think about that: would I have made different choices? To be honest, I say yes, as long as I end up in the same place I am now.

But those broken bits are aspects I have not forgotten. I seek to learn and grow from them, and they help me make better choices here and now, today.

I'm still learning so much about how to love and be real and authentic and compassionate. I'm still learning how not to be judgmental about myself.

Having a near death experience doesn't make you enlightened.

In fact, it can leave you kind of messed up and bumbling along even more than before, because you're straining against a reality that is just not as real as what you touched on. And yet, that one feels both as far away as the horizon and as near as the next movement of your heart. So, it's complicated and it's simple.

Pat: It makes total sense. I was flying one day. I used to fly high performance sailplanes, and I was at 17,000 feet or so over Tahoe, and below was the beautiful aquamarine water. My plane had a fifty-foot wingspan. At the end was a little winglet that was maybe ten or twelve inches tall. And I banked the plane, balanced the entire plane on that little winglet, and that little winglet balanced on a bubble of air. And I rode that bubble of air up through the sky with the sun streaming through the cockpit and the blue waters below, in that incredibly endless blue sky. It was a moment of total endless connection.

It was one of those moments. It was transcendent, it was timeless. It was ephemeral. It is something that has always stuck with me in terms of a greater reality. And it was just a bare taste; just barely touched the surface of what that reality might be.

David: Oh but look at the beautiful symbolism in that; you were sustained, lifted up, made buoyant by this invisible force. And what it required was for you not to use the strength of your huge wings, but to balance on the tip and find that point of vulnerability and connection. It was about letting go of the big control in order to tap into an intuitive control and soar.

Pat: And I soared. I think that's what the sport was about for me; managing invisible updrafts of air to get from point A to point B. And of course, the adventure along the way, but it really was a metaphor for life. There are all these invisible sources of lift. Can you identify them? Can you connect with them? Can you work with them? Can you get to where you want go? And your destination may change.

David: Now, cancer tunes us into that. Cancer can become fuel to lift us higher. Suddenly everything feels different, and where we want to place our energy, there's a priority shift. And most of the time they shift to relationships, the need to be honest about them, and your own humanity, to repair what you can and to let go of what you can't. The wisdom to know the difference, as the prayer says, and to let yourself not need to be good or perfect, but to be real, authentic, and fully awake to the simple moment that you have.

Pat: Perfection is greatly overrated.

David: Yes, and don't let great get in the way of good. Perfection can sabotage our ability to just relax into life, lean into it, and balance on the tip.

Pat: You said something in your book. I don't have the quote in front of me right now, but about how any creative effort really starts with destruction.

David: Yeah. Every act of creation is first an act of destruction. I know that's not encouraging.

We fear things falling apart, and yet mindful presence wakes us up to

the reality that every moment falls apart, every moment passes away, all things change and go with that flow.

That enables you then to identify what you can do, what you need to do. You're not clinging to illusions. You're not trying to control outcomes. You may have your goals, certainly very important, but you work wisely with what is and let things fall apart in order that new things may be created. How much better to be a participant in that instead of resisting it?

How can we use cancer as fuel for that type of vision, dreaming, intuitive creative passion? How can we use it to be more real; more true to ourselves and others?

Pat: I think it's an opportunity to let go of what isn't working, to let go of your emotional armor, to forge a new path, but it is difficult, and it takes courage. There will be many, many bumps in the road if that is a path that you choose.

David: I know that path well, and one of the most important tools for me to continue walking it is a really good sense of humor about myself. I find it hilarious how frequently I trip myself up, how I bumble along through life. And I find that if I can't laugh at that, I become judgmental about it. With that judgmental self-perception, we end up recycling the critical messages about ourselves. That's just an illusion. That's not who we are.

Pat: What advice would you give to somebody facing a significant bump in the road?

David: It's a way for us to realize that we don't need to believe everything we think. We don't need to be controlled by everything we feel. I'm having these thoughts and feelings. They may be difficult at the moment, but they're temporary. And simply by stepping back and observing my thoughts and feelings helps me realize I do have agency here. I do have choice.

As powerful as these thoughts and feelings are, I can just step back and observe them. And in that, I'm more than halfway home, back to my heart.

Reach out for support. Don't think you need to be a hero.

I say that because for most of the patients that I see, the number one concern on their heart is the well-being and emotional peace of their family and loved ones. So, they protect their family from this inner new reality, but in doing so, and I did this, we put on a mask, we try to say, "I'm okay."

They don't need you to do that. They need to be on the same page as you, and to walk the journey with you.

Pat: One of the things that you mentioned in your book that certainly resonated very deeply with me was how we really must change our lives for health and wellbeing. Would you like to talk about that just a little bit?

David: Oh yes. We have so much choice and ability to do that. Let's recognize that we live in a culture that is blessed with such technology and comfort and abundance. There is less poverty and less starvation now than ever before. It feels like there's crises everywhere, but the world is actually in much better shape than it ever has been. Yet, the rate of acceleration of technology and pollution and environmental damage, all of that is spreading, too. So, in this world, we have great choices to lead a healthy life. And it really starts with the basics: exercise, diet, and sleep, the tripod of health. Eating mostly plants, having a good night's sleep (seven to eight hours), and being regularly active.

These three things are monumental in improving the quality of life. And especially when you combine that with good, healthy relationships. We have great choices in changing those foundational aspects of life. And that's the best place to start.

We are not powerless in the face of anything, and as much as we're bombarded with bad news and crises, let's focus upon what we do have control over. Over 50% of cancers are preventable; they're the result of lifestyle choices. So, this is not asking, "Why did I get cancer? Is it because I did this or that?"

If you perseverate upon that, it's gonna be very disempowering. Instead, you can say, "Well I have cancer, what can I do about it? Well, how about let's focus on diet, what can I do there?"

Exercise, even if you've never exercised, just walking, moving twenty minutes to the point that you sweat, is a great thing.

It's all about consistency and how you can be more compassionate and wiser with your thoughts and feelings. How can you be true to yourself and follow your heart?

This is where patient empowerment really starts and needs to be focused on. Don't just be a pin cushion. Don't be at the mercy of the very remarkable medical system and the technology, but work with that foundation of your body, your mind, and your soul in regards to learning:

How do I love?

This is so accessible, and it can happen right now with your next thought, your next thought about yourself. The next thing you put in your mouth, or sitting on the couch playing a video game or whatever, or getting up and going for that walk in the sunshine, getting some vitamin D. It sounds simple. It even sounds naive. It's surprising how few people do it.

Pat: How does all of this impact spirituality in a more global sense?

David: That's a powerful and important question.

In the West, we too often think that spirituality is an individual aspect of our autonomy and who we are as individuals. That's always the emphasis on self in the West, but

spirituality by its definition is a communal thing.

It's all about relationships. It's all about connection, because fundamentally we all arise from the one consciousness. You cannot practice your spirituality in private. It's impossible; it's an oxymoron. It is lived out in your relationship with others and to the environment. It must be manifest in the world.

So globally, I'm excited because I think that we are on the edge of something transformative and monumental. Perhaps even a new spiritual age in which people of all ethnicities and belief systems are focusing upon love and compassion, married to justice and action.

I know that may sound pie in the sky to some of our listeners. And I agree things are probably going to get worse or crazier before they get better. But perhaps as part of a global quickening, something new is being born. Let's not waste the crisis. There is more awareness and knowledge of our place in the universe. More wonder and excitement about where we can go as a species, but we all need to participate in that.

Questions For You to Ponder

How does being judgmental diminish the quality of your life?

How has perfectionism impacted the social, emotional, or spiritual quality of your life?

How might your adversity empower you?

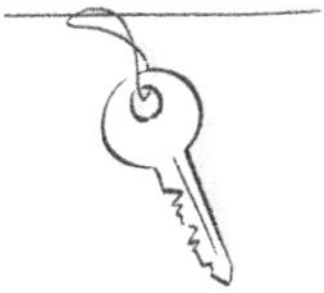

Key Takeaways

- Be real and fully awake to the simple moment you have
- Don't let the great get in the way of the good
- It's ultimately all about love

Five Steps to an Authentic and Meaningful Life

CHAPTER SIXTEEN

The Five Steps

"The Way is not in the sky; the Way is in the heart."

–BUDDHA

I hope you've found themes throughout this book that resonate with you.

These stories speak of courage, hope and resilience. But they go beyond that. They speak to the themes of self-reflection and reclamation, evolution, and even transcendence. They are lessons, large and small, that we can all use in our daily lives.

Effie Parks's story speaks to the power of courage to change one's perceptions. As she challenged her own beliefs and expectations about motherhood, her world opened to even greater love and connection. Her day-to-day life continued to demand perseverance. With newfound insight and compassion, she found a purpose to address her needs and the needs of others in a similar situation.

For Chris Dahl-Bredine, an avalanche made him pause and question how he was living his life. With time to reflect, he decided to chase his dreams to create a new reality that resonated deeply with his soul. Chris's story speaks to the courage to pursue authenticity and purpose in his life.

For Darryll Stinson, a desire to fit in set his life spiraling on a tangent away from his authentic self. But he reclaimed his life and set off on a path to share the wisdom he had learned. Darryll's story speaks to the importance of building our identity from within, rather than from without, and the incredible courage it takes to do so.

All these stories speak to the resilience of the human soul. You have that quality too. You will be tested by life; you will come through it. The key is to find meaning in the bumps along the way.

As I look back at my own life, I see my flying days as a pivotal point with lessons about dependence, interdependence, learning, experience, connection, and community. It was a lesson about reaching high, persevering, and literally learning to soar. It took persistence for me to learn to fly and so much courage for me to take that first flight with Whiskey Oscar. But by being willing to step well outside of my comfort zone, I redefined my life. Soaring was an experience and a metaphor that had a profound impact on me.

From cancer I explored my mind and spirit. Facing my own mortality, I was forced to confront the sometimes shallowness of my own life. Cancer stripped away the superfluous and simplified day-to-day living, enriching my life enormously. It started me on a journey within. That has been and continues to be the most important journey of my life. I can tell you firsthand, it takes courage to go on a quest to know and understand oneself.

I learned about authenticity when I realized that the wonderful material world I had created was built upon an unsustainable foundation void of any true nurture. In solo travel, I was able to further explore my soul and reconnect with my own creativity that had been put aside over the years. Throughout all my journeys, slowly, I built a deep connection with something greater than myself, in nature and in spirit.

As I look back at it all, and as I reflect on the amazing people from my podcast, five steps emerge to finding a life of greater authenticity, value, and meaning. These steps are not linear. They flow into each other; sometimes moving in tandem, sometimes apart.

Each step is about looking within for the change and truth that you seek. Each is a tool to take on all your life's journeys. Additional tools for these five steps are found in the workbook, accessed via the QR code below and found at BumpInTheRoad.us/Readers-Portal. Please check this out. It is an integral part of this book.

CHAPTER SEVENTEEN

Step One: Pivoting Your Perspective

"Life is a balance of holding on and letting go."

–RUMI

Our beliefs define our very reality. When our beliefs fail us, we are forced to pivot and create new perspectives.

With one foot in the past and one moving into the future, you will find yourself in a unique place in time where there is enormous opportunity for personal growth. It's a chance to redefine parts of your life and move forward into a truth that resonates with you.

Sometimes this change is radical. Sometimes not. But in either case, think of it as the universe's way of tapping you on the shoulder. Name the event: Divorce, illness, isolation, parenthood, social rejection, loss—whatever the event—*the problem isn't the problem*. The problem is your perspective and reaction to it. It's a bump in the road telling you that it's time to bring new energy into your life and open your world to new possibilities.

When my ex left for a new job, in a new city, with a new wife, and even a new dog, with hardly a discussion, I was beyond devastated. I wallowed in self-sorrow for quite some time. But the problem wasn't really the divorce and all that ensued. The problem, and the resolution to it, was within me. How would I choose to respond? As a victim? (I did for a while). In justifiable anger? (I tried that too). Or could I see this as an opening to a greater life of my own choosing?

I faced so many bumps. My health, isolation, loss of loved ones, re-defining an entire life. But along the way I discovered courage, hope and resilience. Somewhere during this period, I came to view my life as an adventure. And that is the reality I experienced.

The key to a pivot is to accept the event. You cannot change it, but you can reflect upon it and use it to gain greater self-knowledge. What did you learn about yourself? What are you proud of and what would you do differently? How can you use that self-wisdom to guide your reactions and make better decisions for your future? What traits or beliefs would you like to leave behind? Sometimes ridding yourself of your past allows your future to open in ways you might not expect.

Pivots are emotional and experiential and can be very demanding. For many of us trained to follow society's linear paths, these experiences challenge dearly held beliefs. A successful pivot is ultimately about our willingness to entertain and embrace perspectives outside of our rote comfort zone. It's about taking those first, tentative baby steps and having the courage to persevere. It's about movement, even when we don't know where we're going.

Erik Weihenmayer spent years being lost, isolated, and angry over his loss of sight. When he made a conscious choice to "leave the sighted world behind" he was able to move forward, climb Everest, and so much more. His loss of sight was the event. The very difficult personal decision to accept it and move ahead was the pivot.

Tama Kieves realized that she had to follow her heart, rather than "waste" her time in a prestigious corporate law job. This went against everything society dictated and all that her family valued. She created her pivot when she decided to follow her soul.

Mary Neal tried to deny the reality of her near-death experience. It challenged her scientific world view to its core. But what emerged was a spiritual paradigm shift from hope to trust. Those four words—*from hope to trust*—are a remarkable change in perspective. It took courage to strip away her scientific beliefs to open to a more encompassing possibility.

Seeing the gift in a pivotal event can be slow in coming. We work our way through events, step by step. It takes time and courage to question the perceptions and beliefs that have guided our lives. But once we see through them, they vanish! Poof! Gone! Suddenly a world of possibility opens before us.

It's akin to believing that the Earth is flat. Then a discovery changes that "fact." Suddenly, the fear of falling off the edge of the Earth is gone. The world opens. New lands can be discovered. The same can happen for you.

A pivot is a space that allows us—sometimes forces us—to strip away the behaviors, thoughts, and perceptions that are no longer working and to seek a more authentic path. And the way to do that is to go on a quest for authenticity.

Additional tools for these five steps are found in the workbook, accessed via the QR code below and found at BumpInTheRoad.us/Readers-Portal/

CHAPTER EIGHTEEN

Step Two: Finding Your Authentic Self

Whatever lifts the corners of your mouth, trust that.

–RUMI

Sometimes an event plants a seed that may take years to come to fruition, especially if it contradicts your world as you have known it. Societal and family rules and expectations may clash with what your intuition says. Go to school, get that job, get married. But what if that isn't working for you?

A material world that celebrates the accumulation of titles and "stuff" may be trumped by a more heart-felt desire to create, rather than acquire. How do you explain to your parents who supported you through school and beyond that you want to follow another path? How do you tell your husband or wife that this isn't the life you want?

Seldom are these pivots quick or easy. They often involve prolonged periods of dissatisfaction with no clear answer as to what comes next. Other times they are abrupt, leaving chaos in their wake. But when you truly connect with your authentic self, barriers will fall and a path will appear.

Daring to develop your own unique authenticity is like peeling back the layers of an onion. I must warn you that stripping away the "rules" of your life can be terrifying. But it's also liberating. Our identities are often built on beliefs and behaviors inherited from our families and institutions, none of which may align with who we really are. When we find alignment, life flows.

An example of your roles might include your profession, your role as a parent, or your place in your family. Chances are you are "programmed" with certain responses in each role.

Our behaviors are largely subconscious. Like driving a well-known route in your car, it's easy to tune out. That's when our subconscious takes over. Think about how you react to a difficult situation. Why do you react that way? Where does that behavior really come from?

What were you told as a child? Were you told you were smart or not-so-smart? That you would be a lawyer or doctor? Were you a "good" kid or a "bad" one? As a child, chances are you absorbed parts of that external story, creating a fictional world that made total sense to you at the time and allowed you to meet the expectations of those around you. But was that story true?

Truth lies in the willingness to explore within, to come to terms with the stories we tell ourselves and to release what does not serve us. As you release those outdated beliefs, you'll feel lighter and energized. You'll gain a new perspective. Consider what brings you heart-felt purpose and joy. Consider what makes you smile. Dare to explore what resonates with your soul.

My soul propelled me forward, even as I took many detours along the way. For me, people-pleasing and self-doubt hampered me for years. And perhaps most limiting was that day at the intersection in Connecticut. I stepped away from my authentic self when I built my mental box for a limited life. That disconnect meant that everything was doomed to fail. And fail it did.

My subsequent attempts to reconnect with myself took numerous paths. In that pursuit, there was no right or wrong, just experience. Flying was in part a reaction to all the years that I lived constrained by a limited life. It was a statement of freedom and adventure. It was a portal to wisdom, beauty, and spirit that deeply touched my soul.

Flying provided the catalyst to propel me forward. I moved from the East Coast to the West and, suddenly single, I set out to create my perfect house. It was a multiyear project of acquisitions and renovations. Every item had a story, and I was always on the hunt for that next perfect, quirky piece.

But my outward materialism was really a reflection of my own inner quest for beauty, creativity, and meaning, which I had sidestepped for far too long. I decorated my outer world rather than look too closely at my inner one. I had been defined by my education that implied a strong, driven professional. I had been defined by a limiting illness. I had been defined by divorce and rejection that left a gaping hole in my identity as a valuable person.

On the upside, I also defined myself by my competence and courage as a pilot. I was a fearless traveler, willing to take off cross-country solo, both in the air and on the ground. Flying was a metaphor for a soulful life of astonishing adventure and beauty.

When a diagnosis of supposedly incurable lymphoma came along, time stopped. I became still. All the possessions in the world didn't matter. My net worth had no value. Many of my social circles were equally meaningless. I discovered that what did matter for me was to live a life rich with purpose, beauty, and joy.

Joy was found in the smallest things; the hummingbirds in the garden; the warmth of the sun as I sat in the hammock; the simple delight of being alive. Meditation brought a profound stillness and bliss that I was able to take with me, every day, everywhere

I went. I found myself learning a new language of emotion and spirituality that did not fit into a linear world.

I slowly found purpose in the six years of cancer treatments. I dug deep into my skill toolbox to resurrect my passion for writing and creating. My confidence was still suffering from the ghosts in my head that told me I wasn't good enough, that I didn't matter, and that I had no voice. It took me years to strip away those voices from the past and find confidence in myself and my abilities.

Slowly, very slowly, they crumbled as I wrote, traveled, and photographed my way around the world. And I even won a few awards along the way.

Everyone in this book found a path to their own unique authenticity. Nick Adkins went from corporate warrior to kilt-clad giver of PinkSocks. Jesse Cody found peace, meaning, and his life purpose in the outdoors. Mary Neal found new meaning in a spiritual experience she could not deny.

What are your values? Your attributes? Have the courage to search for your truth. It's an emotional and soulful experience. It will open the door to knowing and loving yourself. It will open the door to finding your personal authenticity.

But to find your authentic self, you must learn to let go.

Additional tools for these five steps are found in the workbook, accessed via the QR code below and found at BumpInTheRoad.us/Readers-Portal/

CHAPTER NINETEEN

Step Three: Release, Rewrite and Rebuild

"The definition of insanity is doing the same thing over and over and expecting different results."

–MARK TWAIN

No one has a perfect life. Everyone has some energy from their past that is limiting their evolution into their future. That energy needs to change, and change, for me, has been most successful when it employs both body and mind. I think of it as release, rewrite, and rebuild.

Our patterns of trauma are stored like memories in our bodies, and they subconsciously guide our response, much like a Pavlovian dog. Eckhardt Tolle calls it the pain body. Joe Dispenza has a meditation-oriented methodology for releasing pain (I find his work to be brilliant). Counseling is another option. Different people respond to different methodologies, but first you need to sense, deep down, that something isn't right. Something is blocking your energy.

Did you have a parent that didn't value you? A teacher that shamed you? Someone that abandoned you? All these events create an emotional experience that settles into your body and psyche, blocking your path forward. You may not even be aware of these obstacles. But when you release these blocks, your energy flows and you've opened energetic space to consciously create something new and better in your life. It's absolutely transformative.

There are many ways to learn to release these thought patterns. I personally seek methodologies in neuropsychology that link your emotions with their physical counterpart. You must recognize and then unlearn those emotional patterns that are mindlessly driving your behavior. Practices like meditation allow you to objectively view your thoughts. Once you can separate yourself from them, you create the power of choice.

For me, a meditation practice helped strip away the endless, meaningless chatter of my mind. What remained may not be easily defined, but it is eternal and real; more real than the endless jumble of thoughts and unsought feelings that had previously consumed me.

The rewiring of my brain has been partly intentional, partly unintentional. Six years of on-again off-again chemo impacted my ability to do complex linear functions, closing down those familiar neuropathways that I had always depended on. Simultaneously, a meditation practice was forming new associations in my brain. Neuroplasticity, the ability of our brains to rewire themselves, is well established. Learning to relearn allows you to view and respond to the world through a new lens. How do you choose to tell your story?

Daring to rewrite our stories gives us such great power. The mental flexibility to see our lives from various points of view means that we are making a conscious choice about how we experience life. What does your story look like told from a perspective of anger? What does it look like from a perspective of gratitude? Can you reframe your story in several different ways and then choose which one you want to live by? (See the online workbook for guidance on this.)

Over the years, I've rewritten the story of my divorce several times. At first, I was abandoned. Discarded. And oh-so-hurt. For years (decades, I hate to admit) the energy of that rejection lingered in my body and my psyche. I told myself it was my get-out-of-jail-free card. But that explanation wasn't owning my own power. And until I found a way to tell my story, to *own* my story, I couldn't rid myself of the hurt.

Then, one day, it struck me. I had used my curiosity to link together some very random events which led me from the East Coast to the West and back again, from one airfield to another, and ultimately to Tahoe. And I didn't just learn to fly; I flew with the "Sky Gods!" I dared to travel with Whiskey Oscar, to pursue a path well outside my comfort zone, and I ultimately stationed her at Minden, Nevada, one of the best places in the world to soar.

And from there, my soaring education continued. I cruised the sky, soaring over mountain ranges, lakes, and desert. I experienced a deep connection with a power greater than myself; a power that was full of joy, beauty, and humility. I did that!

That iteration of my story had nothing to do with divorce. It had nothing to do with hurt or rejection. It had only to do with me. And I finally had to laugh! Only I could connect the diverse dots that led me to such an esoteric sport and all the adventures that followed. My curiosity, creativity, perseverance, and my deep appreciation of beauty had drafted a story uniquely my own.

Reframing our stories implies change, and change is incredibly difficult for most of us. It challenges our habits, our internal dialogue, and our belief systems. It means leaving behind the comfort of the known for the uncertainty of the unknown. The key is finding the energy to take that first step.

Mustering that initial energy is everything. It may be the hardest step you ever take, and you may not understand the significance of it for years to come. You just have to trust that it is your unique path, and it will take you where you need to go. Just remember, it's not a linear trip! It is truly the adventure of a lifetime. Your lifetime.

Change sometimes comes quickly. Sometimes it comes more slowly and requires cultivation. Take the example of committing to a healthier diet.

Because food holds so many associations for all of us, the best chance for sustainable change is most likely incremental. What if you introduced one new healthy food each week? You can keep all your favorite foods. Just try one new thing, say Swiss chard. Make it three ways this week. If you like it, keep it. If not, you never have to have it again. Next week, butternut squash. Or asparagus.

Week by week you are building new experiences, keeping the ones you like and discarding the rest. You're creating a habit of curiosity and change. In six months, you've experimented with twenty-six new foods. If you adopt just half of them, you've created a healthier life. Change that once seemed daunting has become manageable.

Another example. After surgery there is often a period of physical therapy designed to rebuild and strengthen muscles. Day by day, exercise by exercise, you regain your strength. Some days it may seem hard, but you find the energy for just that day. In several months, your body has redefined itself to overcome the trauma of the surgery. By introducing your energy into the situation, you are crafting a new, stronger body.

The same incremental methodology applies to building any new habit. Perhaps you want to learn to meditate. There is a brilliant book, *Eight Minute Meditation: Quiet Your Mind, Change Your Life* by Victor Davich. He takes the reader through a different type of meditation each week. You get to sample a wide range of techniques until you find what resonates for you. He just asks for eight minutes each day. Over time, you're both experimenting with new ideas and building a new habit.

All it takes is the energy and commitment to dare to take that first baby step. It's just a baby step; you can do it. And once you get started, subsequent steps become easier and easier.

Part of rebuilding after a bump is to find gratitude and wisdom in the experience. Gratitude is powerful. It's about seeing the good and living in psychological abundance. It shifts the narrative from 'why is this happening to me' to 'why is this happening for me.' Gratitude will make you happy.

When I look back at my divorce, I am so grateful for it. Being expelled from my tribe hurt deeply. But in retrospect, I can see what a nightmare it would have been to be stuck in that quagmire. While the pain was very real, it opened my world for much-needed personal growth and exploration.

But before growth comes what I call "the muck;" that place where the world looks dark and unchangeable. It's a place void of gratitude. It's where we fall back on all our past emotional and behavioral programming to cope with the situation.

Rather than releasing what is no longer serving us and looking ahead, we are stuck. We experience our bump through the backward-looking lens of the past. We react, sometimes without much awareness. But as we become more aware of our habitual patterns of behavior, we can choose to change them.

What if we could actively watch our thoughts form and consciously choose both our thoughts and response? What if we could learn to understand what drives us?

That's where the mind game comes into play.

Additional tools for these five steps are found in the workbook, accessed via the QR code below and found at BumpInTheRoad.us/Readers-Portal/

CHAPTER TWENTY

Step Four: The Mind Game

Keep silent because the world of silence is a vast fullness.

–RUMI

This is an old Zen story. There are numerous versions. Here is one:

Once, a long time ago, there was a wise Zen master. People from far and near would seek his counsel and ask for his wisdom. Many would come and ask him to teach them, enlighten them in the way of Zen. He seldom turned anyone away.

One day an important man, a man used to commanding others, came to visit the master. "I have come today to ask you to teach me about Zen. Open my mind to enlightenment."

The tone was on of an important man used to getting his own way.

The Zen master smiled and said that they should discuss the matter over a cup of tea. When the tea was served the master poured his visitor a cup. He poured and he poured, and the tea rose to the rim and began to spill over the table and finally onto the robes of the wealthy man. Finally, the visitor shouted, "Enough. You are spilling the tea all over. Can't you see the cup is full?"

The master stopped pouring and smiled at his guest. "You are like this teacup, so full that nothing more can be added. Come back to me when the cup is empty. Come back to me with an empty mind."

Emptying one's mind doesn't mean visiting a silent retreat in an exotic locale for a month or more. It's an entirely learnable skill that will change your life and your world. Once you experience silence, you will be able to see how busy your mind typically is. It's like any set of contrasts. You can't understand hot until you know cold; darkness until you know light; peace until you know turmoil.

Learning to quiet your mind allows you to become a witness to the stream of thoughts that seem to be constantly present. Mental to do lists, worries, and imaginary fears can be seen for what they are: distractions of your ego and imagination.

Your mind conjures up all sorts of things that never come true or are detrimental to your well-being. Your mind may tell you that you're fat, you're ugly, you're not worthy, you failed to do this or tha t. . . name your diatribe. We all have them. We all need to still them.

There are many approaches to finding stillness. Some practices focus on breath; some on mantras; some on a fixed object. Some people find that sound is their opening to a quiet mind. There is no right or wrong. It's all about what works for you. Experiment and play. Stillness is an essential asset for building a conscious life.

The magic that comes with a quiet mind opens into a timeless, endless place of immense presence. It's a stark contrast to the limitations imposed by the "monkey mind."

"Monkey mind" is a Buddhist phrase that describes the never ending, repetitive, and judgmental jumble of thoughts that babble through the brain. Your thoughts, like the full teacup, do not allow for new patterns of living and learning. Your thoughts actually limit your perspective, and thus your experience. You can choose to live a much more expanded life.

An empty mind expands your world.

You are no longer limited by the voice in your head. Like the gentleman in the Zen story who is told to return when his tea cup is empty, a quiet mind opens the door to new possibilities. The deep peace that comes with this practice becomes part of you. Road rage? A thing of the past. Impatience in the grocery line? Gone. Mental peace will change your world. Tom Cronin's story about a bond trader turned meditation master is a great example of this.

Mastering your mind is perhaps one of the most profound skills you can learn. It is nothing short of life-changing. But creating change, like learning any new skill, takes practice and persistence, even when you think there is no time to devote to such pursuits.

In the meditation community there is a saying: "If you don't have time to meditate for an hour, meditate for two," suggesting that putting peace and presence at the forefront of your agenda is of the utmost importance. It is so important because:

You will learn to live more fully in the present when you become present.

It seems so simple, yet the impact is so profound. With presence, there is no past or future. There is only this moment. And this moment is endlessly deep and rich with the experience of being alive.

For just one day, make stillness your focus. Between your thoughts there's a space. It's quiet in that space. Find it. Stay with it as long as you can. Find it again. Experience it. Would you like to have this peace be a part of your life?

The mind game is a lifelong pursuit for greater awareness. It will help you become more present and will free you from being a reactive slave to your emotional and social programming. It will help you find perspective and opportunity, even in difficult times. It will bring you peace.

In short, it will change your life because in the silence, you can start to sense your unique purpose.

Additional tools for these five steps are found in the workbook, accessed via the QR code below and found at BumpInTheRoad.us/Readers-Portal/

CHAPTER TWENTY-ONE

Step Five: Your Unique Purpose

"Your purpose in life is to find your purpose and give your whole heart and soul to it."

–BUDDHA

Finding purpose starts with getting in touch with your authentic self. Our purpose may change with time. As we evolve and grow, we have an opportunity to discard what we no longer need and be open to new experiences and wisdom.

In exploring your unique purpose, be curious, open yourself to new possibilities, and pursue what touches you. If it doesn't suit you, discard it. Have courage. Be adventurous.

Also pay attention to your programmed responses and thought patterns that do not benefit you. Don't be hemmed in by what your mother, father, sister, teacher, boss, or ex said about you. Listen to your heart and inner guidance. Know that you are infinitely valuable and there is great wisdom within you. Trust that wisdom to guide you in your search.

And what is it we're all searching for? Joseph Campbell speculated that what we're looking for isn't meaning but the deep, intense, transcendental *experience* of being alive. We're looking for that experience that speaks to our timeless soul but is rooted in the here and now.

Such an experience is often referred to as "flow." It's where challenge, ability, and focus meet to create an optimal and even transcendental experience. In the classic book *Flow: The Psychology of Optimal Experience*, Mihaly Csikszentmihalyi talks about optimal experience, where one's focus is so intense that everything else falls away. It's like entering a different dimension of space and time. It's completely immersive. Time slows. Everything is now.

Sports such as rock climbing, high-altitude mountaineering, soaring, and sailing are all examples of flow. So are knitting, writing, cooking, art, walking, hiking, and any other activity you can think of.

Think of flow as a meditation of doing where you are one with the universe of creativity and possibility.

So how do you experience flow? And how is it connected to your unique purpose?

Purpose is about being one with your heart and soul. Flow is about presence, competence, and challenge. Together, purpose plus flow offer a transcendental experience. It is total immersion in what Joseph Campbell called the experience of being alive.

I found flow soaring. It was part of the utter addiction of the sport. But to get to that state took time and the development of competency. I followed my heart, but I still had to learn to fly, transition into more complex planes, and practice, practice, practice. Flying was my purpose. Flow was the hard-earned confluence of my skills meeting the magic of the Earth and the sky, along with the great privilege of being part of it all.

Flow can be experienced anywhere, any time. It's about exploring the depths of our creativity in a timeless space created by our own awareness. It's about both inhabiting the present and the eternal simultaneously.

Flow is an experience, a state of mind, and a state of being.

I think of flow as soulful energy manifesting itself where you are one with your why, aligned with your authentic self, where nothing exists but that one timeless moment, forever.

One of my favorite quotes about being in the flow comes from mountaineer Erik Weihenmayer. Erik, although blind, had conquered Everest and the Seven Summits, but navigating the Colorado River rapids required a different sort of skill; a skill of trust, of letting go and becoming one with the river. Eight years of training to kayak the river led him to this realization:

Climbing was more about bringing yourself forth, asserting your will over an extreme, inhospitable environment. Yet trying to apply that learning to rivers had failed. Perhaps, the secrets of a river were not revealed by trying to exert the ego over it, but rather by letting go and allowing the river to consume you, all the way down to the core, by simply giving in to the unknowable and writing music you would never hear. By surrendering, it allowed the river to erode everything and wash away the crust, until there was nothing left but that inner light. . . Unencumbered, that light was free to flow out and fuse with the landscape, with the energy of the unstoppable river. Maybe this was as close as we could ever get to understanding, just a brief portal flash of that light connecting with something bigger, something mysterious and infinite."

–From No Barriers: A Blind Man's Journey To Kayak The Grand Canyon, Erik Weihenmayer with permission from St. Martin's Press

From conquering mountains to moving with and becoming part of the cadence of the river is a massive shift in perspective. That shift opened him to the spiritual dimension of being in the flow and that exquisite connection to something "bigger, mysterious, and infinite."

That connection with the infinite lives beyond our bodies and minds, but within us. Finding our "why" opens the door to a purpose that is greater than ourselves and connects us with the world of spirit, wisdom, and energy.

Use your strengths to find your unique purpose. Have the courage to trust yourself. Stick with it. You're smart. You're capable. Take that chance. It will lead to a path that will define your life in a way that is true to you and congruent with your soul. It will take you to amazing places.

Additional tools for these five steps are found in the workbook, accessed via the QR code below and found at BumpInTheRoad.us/Readers-Portal/

CHAPTER TWENTY-TWO

Putting it All Together

"I take to the open road. Healthy, free, the world before me."

–WALT WHITMAN

I have come to see life as a road trip, full of bumps, potholes, and extraordinary views. Sometimes you get lost. Sometimes that's good, sometimes not. But it's all about the journey and what we learn along the way.

It's about adopting and cultivating a mindset that allows your strengths to shine. Your strengths might be love, kindness, or teamwork. For me, curiosity, creativity, and beauty are driving forces. For all of us, it's about scripting your own unique story, moment by moment. Over time, the tapestry of life starts to make sense, and with greater wisdom we tell our stories and we evolve.

Our stories are powerful. We tell our tales as humans do, with wandering prose, with starts and stops. We tell our stories with emotion, not knowing the end. And we experience the wisdom of our stories only in retrospect.

We may waffle as we struggle to find our way. But the key is to look beyond the specifics of the story; to look to the deeper lessons that are relevant to all of us and do not change with time. Those are the lessons that teach us. Growth comes from within, from self-reflection, and from making conscious choices.

When you hit a bump in the road:

Shift Your Perspective

A bump, by its very nature, sends you careening off-road. Don't panic. Don't project a dire future. Chances are you'll come to rest with a few dings and scrapes. You will be okay.

Take a deep breath. Again. There are numerous breathing exercises that can help ground you. Breath can be a portal to calming your body and your mind.

I once had a friend that had a questionable mammogram. She spent the next two weeks convinced she was going to go through chemo, lose her hair, and possibly die. She was on the ceiling, stressing, and chasing down every negative thought that came into her mind. Thankfully, none of this came true. The tests came back fine.

What might she have done? She might have simply focused on gratitude for the moment. She might have explored her need for control and her reactions to that uncertainty. She might have asked herself if she was living the life she wanted. Was she true to herself? How were her relationships with others? Given the chance, what might she change?

The lesson is that there are numerous ways to approach an issue. The problem isn't the problem. The problem lies in your reaction. Ask yourself, what is the lesson in the situation? What do you need to learn? That simple question—"What do I need to learn?"—can revolutionize your life.

Part of personal evolution is to consider the lens you are using to view the world. Do you see the world as judging you? Do you see the world as unfriendly? Do you see the world through a prism of rules to be followed? Typically, we project our lens onto the world around us. Your view of the world is really a reflection of yourself. Ask yourself what you're experiencing.

Try seeing the world through a lens of gratitude, awe, or love. Try to see connection and oneness, even where there would seem to be none. Try changing your lens and seeing things anew.

Your Authentic Self

The answers you seek will come from within. Be still and feel. Because the way through any life event is not linear or intellectual. It's emotional and experiential. The more time you spend peeling away the layers of your own story, seeking your truest self, the more powerful will be the outcome of your bump in the road. Once you are in congruence with yourself, all of life starts to fall in line, even when it doesn't go your way.

Release, Rewrite and Rebuild

The mind and body are interconnected. Our subconscious accounts for 95 percent of our brain activity, yet we are largely unaware of the unconscious programs embedded there. We need to learn to let go of the thoughts and behaviors that do not serve us and to create a path with higher energy. As we recognize our old patterns of programming, we can release them. This is so incredibly powerful. Whether you work with a licensed professional, go to a retreat, or are an avid reader seeking answers, you deserve to let go of the energy that holds you back.

The Mind Game

Learning to quiet your mind is a game changer.

When you experience a quiet mind, you create the opportunity to explore your own psyche in a search for authenticity.

In this space, you can learn to observe your mind and consciously choose your thoughts.

This isn't about affirmations. It's much deeper. It's about becoming aware and making conscious choices. It's about creating your world view in alignment with your soul. If you stay with this quest, you can find profound peace and personal empowerment.

Quieting your mind is one of the most powerful tools for reflection, understanding, and self-compassion. Self-compassion is so important, because until we learn compassion for ourselves, we cannot truly give it to others.

Finding Your Unique Purpose

This is where the fun is! It's not a linear path and there is no right or wrong. It's all about what is right for you at this point in time. A purpose isn't about, say, becoming a doctor. It's much deeper. It's the emotion that lies behind the purpose. Purpose is an emotional force that drives you, not a degree that defines you.

Going through changes in your life, your purpose may also change. But the need for a purpose doesn't. Studies show that people that have a purpose are happier, have a lower risk of death, are more optimistic, and have greater resiliency and hope. Daring to seek your "why" is an act of courage, loving adventure, and satisfaction. Go for it!

Navigating Life's Bumps

Every challenge is truly an opportunity if you make it so. Change can be exciting, because in that gap between the old and the new is unlimited possibility. It's an infinitely creative place where you get to redefine yourself and your world view. What do you choose?

Each of the steps cited above draws on all the stories in this book and is a book unto itself. I've included an extensive list of resources and a workbook that can help you explore these dimensions of finding congruence in your life and with your soul. Finding purpose, experiencing flow, and having inner peace are an amazing part of being alive.

I cannot stress enough that you are the creator of your life. You may not be able to control everything that happens, but you can control your reactions and your perceptions. You create your reality. Somewhere in your bump are soulful lessons that can open new doors if you dare to take that first step into the unknown. And sometimes that first step is to look within.

If there is a call to action in this book, it is to celebrate every moment of your life, embrace your bumps, and live and grow along the way. Become a conscious human, one that is kind. And most of all, have a sense of curiosity, gratitude, and adventure. Because in our adventures lie the best and most meaningful stories.

Reading and Resources

Reading and Resources

I'm an avid reader and I love to share great books. Thus, this list! Many of these people have written multiple books, some of which are not listed here. Be sure to do a web search by the author's name to see if there is anything of interest to you.

Many of these authors also have websites. Some have been guests on the podcast *Bump in The Road*. Explore and see what resonates with you. I'm sure I've overlooked far too many wonderful books, but this is meant to be a starting point for your own explorations.

Psychology

Brown, Brené. 2012. *Daring Greatly: How the Courage to Be Vulnerable Transforms the Way We Live, Love, Parent, and Lead*. London: Penguin Books Ltd.

Csikszentmihalyi, Mihaly. 1990. *Flow: The Psychology of Optimal Experience*. New York: Harper and Row.

Hawkins, David R, and Scott Jeffrey. 2011. *Dissolving the Ego, Realizing the Self: Contemplations from the Teachings of David R. Hawkins, M.D., PH. D.* Carlsbad, Calif.: Hay House.

Spirituality

Alexander, Eben. 2013. *Proof of Heaven: A Neurosurgeon's Journey into the Afterlife*. New York: Simon & Schuster.

Deepak Chopra. 2007. *Seven Spiritual Laws of Success*. San Rafael, Calif.: Amber-Allen; Enfield.

Foundation for Inner Peace. 1992. *A Course in Miracles*. Glen Elen, Ca: Foundation for Inner Peace.

Lesser, Elizabeth. 2008. *The Seeker's Guide: Making Your Life a Spiritual Adventure*. New York: Villard.

Maginley, David. 2016. *Beyond Surviving: Cancer and Your Spiritual Journey*. Halifax, Ns: Tristan Press.

Moorjani, Anita. 2015. *Dying to Be Me: My Journey from Cancer, to Near Death, to True Healing*. Carlsbad, Calif.: Hay House.

Neal, Mary C. 2017. *7 Lessons from Heaven: How Dying Taught Me to Live a Joy-Filled Life*. New York: Convergent Books.

Neal, Mary C. 2012. *To Heaven and Back: A Doctor's Extraordinary Account of Her Death, Heaven, Angels, and Life Again : A True Story*. Colorado Springs, Colo.: Waterbrook Press.

Novels, Biographies, and Other Great Reads

Atwood, Janet Bray, and Chris Attwood. 2009. *The Passion Test: The Effortless Path to Discovering Your Destiny*. London: Pocket.

Coelho, Paulo. 2014. *The Alchemist: 25th Anniversary Edition.* San Francisco: HarperOne.

Frankl, Victor E. (1946) 2006. *Man's Search for Meaning*. Boston: Beacon Press.

Hesse, Hermann. (1922) 2017. *Siddhartha*. Paris: Grasset.

Hari, Johann. 2018. *Lost Connections*. New York: Bloomsbury.

Hari, Johann. 2023. *Stolen Focus*. New York: Crown.

McSally, Martha. 2021. *Dare to Fly: Simple Lessons in Never Giving Up*. New York: WIlliam Morrow.

Mazan, Steve. 2011. *Dying to Do Letterman: Turning Someday into Today*. Deerfield Beach, Fl: Health Communications.

Remen, Rachel Naomi, and Jacqueline M Berg. 2007. *The Little Book of Kitchen Table Wisdom*. New York: Riverhead Books.

Ruiz, Miguel. 1997. *The Four Agreements: A Practical Guide to Personal Freedom*. San Rafael, Calif.: Amber-Allen.

Shapiro, Dani. 2019. *Inheritance*. New York: Anchor Books.

Singer, Michael A. 2016. *The Surrender Experiment: My Journey into Life's Perfection*. London: Yellow Kite.

Singer, Michael A, and Institute of Noetic Sciences. 2013. *The Untethered Soul: The Journey beyond Yourself.* Oakland, Calif.: Noetic Books, Institute of Noetic Sciences, New Harbinger Publications, Inc.

Taylor, Jill Bolte. 2016. *My Stroke of Insight: A Brain Scientist's Personal Journey*. New York: Penguin Books.

Weihenmayer, Erik, and Buddy Levy. 2017. *No Barriers: A Blind Man's Journey to Kayak the Grand Canyon*. New York: Thomas Dunne Books/St. Martin's Press.

The Mind/Body Connection

Braden, Gregg. 2020. *Wisdom Codes: Ancient Words to Rewire Our Brains and Heal Our Hearts*. Carlsbad, Calif.: Hay House.

Dispenza, Joe, and Daniel G Amen. 2015. *Breaking the Habit of Being Yoursel : How to Lose Your Mind and Create a New One*. Carlsbad, Calif.: Hay House.

Dispenza, Joe. 2019. *Becoming Supernatural How Common People Are Doing the Uncommon*. Hay House.

Dispenza, Joe. 2015. *You Are the Placebo: Making Your Mind Matter*. Carlsbad, Calif.: Hay House.

Kolk, Bessel van der. 2014. *The Body Keeps the Score: Mind, Brain, and Body in the Transformation of Trauma*. London: Penguin Books.

Lipton, Bruce H. 2016. *The Biology of Belief: Unleashing the Power of Consciousness, Matter & Miracles*. Carlsbad, Calif.: Hay House.

Miller, Emmett E. 1997. *Deep Healing: The Essence of Mind/Body Medicine*. Carlsbad, Ca: Hay House.

Pert, Candace B. 2003. *Molecules of Emotion*. New York: Scribner.

Siegel, Bernie. 1990. *Peace, Love & Healing*. New York: Harper Perennial.

On Meditation

Cronin, Tom, and Jacqui Fifer. 2020. *The Portal*. Strawberry Hills, N.S.W.: Dyslexic Books.

Davich, Victor N. 2014. *8 Minute Meditation: Quiet Your Mind, Change Your Life*. New York: Perigee.

Dove, Pragito. 2020. *Lunchtime Enlightenment: Expressive Meditations for Manifesting Peace, Prosperity, and Passion*. Cortaro, Az: Dove Publishing.

Kabat-Zinn, Jon. 2004. *Wherever You Go, There You Are*. London: Piatkus.

Rosenthal, Norman E. 2012. *Transcendence: Healing and Transformation through Transcendental Meditation*. New York: Jeremy P. Tarcher/Penguin.

Shetty, Jay. 2020. *Think like a Monk: How to Train Your Mind for Peace & Purpose Every Day*. New York: Simon & Schuster.

Transforming Your Consciousness

Hay, Louise L. 2017. *You Can Heal Your Life*. Sydney Hay House, Inc.

Hensel, Gary. *I Am*. Bloomington, Ind.: Balboa Press, 2017.

Hensel, Gary. *Lessons For a Spiritual Warrior*. AWOKE Publishing, 2021.

Kieves, Tama. 2018. *Thriving through Uncertainty: Moving Beyond Fear of the Unknown and Making Change Work for You*. New York: Tarcher Perigee.

Orloff, Judith. 2009. *Emotional Freedom: Liberate Yourself from Negative Emotions and Transform Your Life*. New York: Harmony Books.

Tolle, Eckhart. 2004. *The Power of NOW: A Guide to Spiritual Enlightenment*. Vancouver, B.C.: Namaste Pub.; Novato, Calif.: New World Publishing.

Watts, Alan W. 1999. *Way of Zen*. New York: Vintage Books.

Zukav, Gary, Oprah Winfrey, and Maya Angelou. 1989. *The Seat of the Soul*. New York: Simon & Schuster.

Zukav, Gary, and Linda Francis. 2007. *The Heart of the Soul: Emotional Awareness*. New York: Free Press.

Pure Inspiration

Paul Gordon Stoltz, and Erik Weihenmayer. 2010. *The Adversity Advantage: Turning Everyday Struggles into Everyday Greatness: Updated with New Stories from the Seven Summits and Expedition Photographs*. New York: Simon & Schuster.

Siegel, Bernie S, and Andrea Hurst. 2011. *A Book of Miracles: Inspiring True Stories of Healing, Gratitude, and Love*. Novato, Calif.: New World Library.

Weihenmayer, Erik. 2002. *Touch the Top of the World.* Auburn, Ca: Audio Partners C.

Weihenmayer, Erik, and Buddy Levy. 2017. *No Barriers: A Blind Man's Journey to Kayak the Grand Canyon.* New York: Thomas Dunne Books/St. Martin's Press.

Web-Based Resources

There are many web-based programs. This is one resource that offers a fascinating insight into one's strengths.

"VIA Character Strengths Survey & Character Profile Reports." n.d. www.viacharacter.org http://www.viacharacter.org

Bump in the Road Workbook

Or sign in at BumpInTheRoad.us/Readers-Portal/

Sailplane Glossary of Terms

Soaring is a unique sport with its own specialized language. Learning to soar is a combination of mastering a great deal of aviation-related technical information and procedures, and then developing an understanding of the energy in the sky and how to effectively use it. It's about maximizing the capabilities of both the pilot and the aircraft. It is an exhilarating and humbling experience. It is a challenge and an art.

Here are some of the terms scattered through this glossary and through my stories:

Bernoulli's Principle: Daniel Bernoulli was a Swiss mathematician who studied the movement of fluids, like air and water. He realized that the faster the fluid flows, the less pressure it generates.

This applies to aviation in that the upper surface of the wing is curved; the bottom is flat. Air must move more quickly over the upper curved surface of the wing than it does over the bottom. This pressure differential creates lift which allows the wing, and the airplane, to fly.

Center of Gravity-CG (see Weight and Balance): The CG is the point where the aircraft is balanced. It impacts the stability of the aircraft and must fall within specified limits.

Center of Gravity (CG) Hook: This is where the tow rope connects to the sailplane. It is located at the front of the wheel well, under the seat of the pilot, at or near the CG.

Cloud Base: The bottom of the cloud. Clouds form as rising moisture condenses. This makes a cloud a potential indicator for lift.

Cloud formation cycles throughout the day, so you must be aware of what is going on in the sky. Particularly in the American West, rapid cloud formation can lead to massive thunderstorms. You really don't want to fly into a thunderstorm!

Final Approach: This is it. You're coming in to land! No second chances! Remember: Flying is the second greatest thrill known to man. Landing is the first.

Flaps: Positive flaps change the curvature of the wing, resulting in increased drag and lift, allowing the plane to fly more slowly, particularly on final approach.

Whiskey Oscar had both positive and negative flaps. The positive flaps allowed her to make very short field landings. The negative flaps were essentially "warp speed," allowing her to accelerate quickly.

'Floating the flaps" refers to not locking in the flap setting, but gently manually guiding the lever to a point that feels like the optimal configuration for best climb in each circumstance. It took me some time to develop the feel for the plane to have the confidence to do this.

Glide Ratio: The glide ratio determines how far a sailplane can glide. For example, a glide ratio of 40:1 means that the plane can travel forty feet while losing only one foot of altitude. So, at 10,000 feet above the ground, a 40:1 sailplane can travel seventy-five miles assuming still air (no lift or sink).

Longer wings generally translate into higher glide ratios, and thus the ability to travel longer distances without needing to stop to find lift. Thus, a glider with a 70:1 glide ratio could glide 132 miles and would be a good choice for setting long timed distance records. But it's not as responsive or as fun to fly as a fifteen or seventeen-meter plane.

Landing Checklist: This checklist is used to ensure that the plane is properly configured for landing and the pilot is focused on key things.

Mine was UFFSTALL:

- **U**ndercarriage (make sure the gear is down!) You do not want to land with your gear up.
- **F**laps: These should be set to landing configuration (you have many choices here, depending on the length of the landing field and your position relative to your touch down point).
- **F**: The extra "F" is a not-so-gentle reminder that if you f*#!ing stall, you die!
- **S**peed is a critical component. Too fast and your landing could be ugly (although there are times when the weather warrants a faster landing). Too slow and you stall.
- **T**rim: Set the trim at a constant attitude and airspeed to minimize the workload on the pilot during landing
- **A**ltitude: You constantly monitor this both visually and with your instruments to understand where you are relative to the runway.

- **Look out**, watch for other traffic, especially entering the landing pattern!
- **Land**: You want to manage the energy so that you stop off the runway, leaving the way clear for other traffic. Now remember to breathe and know that any landing you walk away from is a good one.

Landing Out: This refers to landing somewhere other than an airport. It occurs when you run out of altitude. Your landing spot may be a farmer's field, an abandoned road, or a dry lake. There are numerous things to consider: obstacles such as power lines, wind direction, wing clearance, condition of the soil, and so much more. In short, it's a pretty stressful situation. And after you land, your flight isn't over. You still have to get the sailplane out of the field, into its trailer, and return home. This is where you find out if you have any friends, and you buy them dinner and lots of beer once you get back safely to the airfield.

Lift: Rising air creates lift. When you find lift, you want to center your plane in it for maximum climb. Lift might come from the formation of a cloud, a mountainside facing the sun, air colliding with a mountain (which may produce wave), or from colliding air masses as in a convergence zone. Sometimes lift just appears as a "blue street," an invisible avenue of lift, with no obvious source. When you find this, just enjoy the ride!

Prohibited Airspace: These are areas over which you may not fly. NOTAMs (Notice to Airmen) may have additional flight restrictions.

Ridge Flying: Ridge flying means soaring orographic lift, which is generated when air is compressed as it moves up over an obstacle such as a ridge, hill, or mountain. This often occurs with the passage of a weather front, and it creates a band of lift just upwind of the ridge. Sailplane pilots carefully study the weather in search for such opportunities.

The good news is that the wind and lift associated with a massive weather front passing through can be steady and reliable. The bad news is that if there is a pause in the wind or a shift in its direction, you need to find a place to land *fast*. Landing out—i.e., not at an airport–is not a low stress experience.

Flying the ridge can be spectacular, particularly over the Appalachian Ridge in the fall. It means low altitude flying close to the terrain to maximize speed. Some pilots say that if you're not knocking the squirrels out of the trees, you're not low enough.

Rotor: Extreme turbulence associated with lenticular clouds and wave flying (See Wave).

Rudder: The rudder provides directional stability in the air and is used to control the yaw of the plane. On the ground, the rudder pedals are used to steer the plane on the runway.

On takeoff, after giving the thumbs up to the ground crew, the pilot presses the rudder pedals back and forth, causing the rudder to waggle. This signals the tow pilot that the sailplane is ready to launch.

Sink: An area of descending air that will carry the sailplane with it. Rule of thumb: Speed up in sink, slow down in lift.

Sheer (Wind Sheer): A rapid change of wind direction or velocity. This disrupts the flow of air over the wing (which is what enables the plane to fly; see Bernoulli's Principle) and can cause a loss of airspeed and/or a stall/spin.

Thermal: A thermal is a rising column of air. "Thermalling" refers to flying in that column of air to gain altitude.

One usually thermals at a fairly steep bank to try to stay centered in the rising air. The key is to find the core of the thermal (the area of lift) and center the plane in the best (rising) air.

Effective thermalling, like all of soaring, is an art.

Trim: A control that sets the attitude and thus the speed of the plane. This means less manual input from the pilot to maintain a constant airspeed and frees the pilot to focus on other aspects of flight, particularly while landing.

Wave: Wave is a meteorological phenomenon often characterized by massive lenticular clouds. It occurs when a weather system meets a mountain range or other such obstacle, creating a broad band of rising air (lift) that can be flown to heights well over 30,000 feet.

Wave flying is spectacular and sometimes more than a little scary. It can be accompanied by dramatic areas of instability and sink, called rotor. Temperatures aloft hover around negative fifty degrees Fahrenheit over 30,000 feet. A compressed oxygen system is required. Dress warmly!

Weight and Balance: This is a critical calculation with lots of math and theory. The bottom line is that the center of gravity (CG) of the aircraft must be within certain limits for safety and control. If it is not, the nose may pitch uncontrollably up or down, making the aircraft potentially uncontrollable. Neither place is where you want to be!

Wheel Dolly: An apparatus that wraps around the rear of the fuselage to facilitate ground handling. Be sure it is removed prior to takeoff.

Wingspan: The length from wingtip to wingtip. The longer the wingspan, the greater the glide ratio.

Acknowledgements

Thanks are due to many people. I'm sure I'm missing many, but special thanks to Sam Harry, the naval aviator who taught me to fly by the seat of my pants; to Dave and Sharon Pixton who were so kind and welcoming at MASA; Jim Meiklejohn; John Hearn, aka Tango One; Tom and Billy Stowers at High Country Soaring; Heinz Weisenbuehler; Monte Sullivan; Rebecca Koch; Wendy Wagner; Stephen Jacobs; and many others along the way.

About the Author

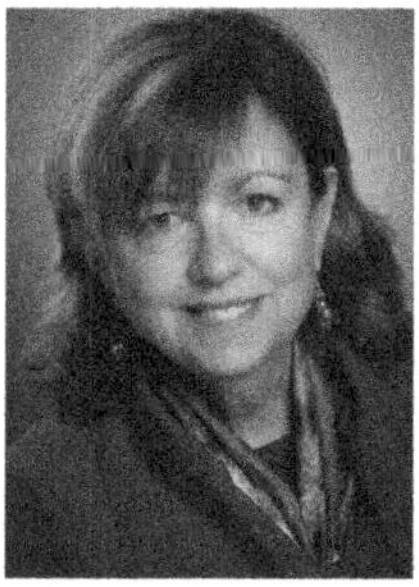

Pat Wetzel graduated from the University of Pennsylvania and Wharton Business School and started her adult life in New York. A serious neurological disease would be her first bump in the road, redefining her life. From there, numerous other bumps propelled her on a quest for meaning and authenticity.

Ms. Wetzel is an award-winning author. You can learn more about her on her website BumpInTheRoad.us. Contact her at talk@BumpInTheRoad.us. She is available for speaking engagements.

Follow Pat on social media:

Facebook: Facebook.com/BumpInTheRd
Twitter : @CancerRoadTrip
Instagram: @CancerRoadTrip

She is also on LinkedIn.

Ms.Wetzel currently lives in Prescott, AZ and is working on a series of *Bump in the Road* books. The next two books scheduled are *Bump in the Road: Strong Women* and *Bump in the Road: Cancer*.

Made in the USA
Monee, IL
14 October 2023

44466294R00149